THE BREAST RECONSTRUCTION GUIDEBOOK

D0376168

KATHY STELIGO

THE BREAST RECONSTRUCTION GUIDEBOOK

Issues and Answers

from Research to Recovery

FOURTH EDITION

JOHNS HOPKINS UNIVERSITY PRESS
Baltimore

Note to the Reader: This book is not meant to substitute for medical care of people with breast cancer, and treatment should not be based solely on its contents. Instead, treatment must be developed in a dialogue between the individual and his or her physician. Our book has been written to help with that dialogue.

Drug dosage: The author and publisher have made reasonable efforts to determine that the selection of drugs discussed in this text conform to the practices of the general medical community. The medications described do not necessarily have specific approval by the U.S. Food and Drug Administration for use in the diseases for which they are recommended. In view of ongoing research, changes in governmental regulation, and the constant flow of information relating to drug therapy and drug reactions, the reader is urged to check the package insert of each drug for any change in indications and dosage and for warnings and precautions. This is particularly important when the recommended agent is a new and/or infrequently used drug.

© 2012, 2017 Johns Hopkins University Press
All rights reserved. Published 2017
First and second editions © 2002, 2005
Kathy Steligo
Printed in the United States of America on acid-free paper
9 8 7 6 5 4 3 2 1

Johns Hopkins University Press
2715 North Charles Street
Baltimore, Maryland 21218-4363
www.press.jhu.edu

LIBRARY OF CONGRESS
CATALOGING-IN-PUBLICATION DATA

Names: Steligo, Kathy, author.
  Title: The breast reconstruction guidebook : issues and answers from research to recovery / Kathy Steligo.
  Description: Fourth edition. | Baltimore : Johns Hopkins University Press, 2017. | Includes bibliographical references and index.
  Identifiers: LCCN 2016044786|
ISBN 9781421422961 (pbk. : alk. paper) |
ISBN 1421422964 (pbk. : alk. paper) |
ISBN 9781421422978 (electronic) |
ISBN 1421422972 (electronic)
  Subjects: LCSH: Mammaplasty—Popular works. | Musculocutaneous flaps—Popular works. | Mammaplasty—Complications—Popular works. | Women—Health and hygiene—Popular works. | Breast—Cancer—Surgery—Popular works. | Breast—Cancer—Patients—Rehabilitation—Popular works.
  Classification: LCC RD539.8 .S73 2017 | DDC 618.1/90592—dc23
  LC record available at https://lccn.loc.gov/2016044786

A catalog record for this book is available from the British Library.

Special discounts are available for bulk purchases of this book. For more information, please contact Special Sales at 410-516-6936 or specialsales@press.jhu.edu.

Johns Hopkins University Press uses environmentally friendly book materials, including recycled text paper that is composed of at least 30 percent post-consumer waste, whenever possible.

Contents

Foreword

Minas Chrysopoulo, MD
PRMA Plastic Surgery Center for Advanced
Breast Reconstruction

Many people mistakenly think that breast reconstruction is merely a cosmetic procedure. It is far more than that. Breast reconstruction can make women whole again after mastectomy or lumpectomy. It restores much of what nature provided but cancer (or the threat of it) has taken away. It is also covered by insurance in the majority of cases, thanks to a 1998 federal mandate.

For many patients, breast reconstruction is also a statement of intent . . . the intention to survive the disease. Although not all women choose to have reconstruction, they should all have the option to make that decision for themselves. Unfortunately, many patients who are facing or who have had mastectomy or lumpectomy are not offered reconstruction. Even when reconstruction is discussed, oftentimes the conversation doesn't include *all* the options.

The breast cancer surgery decisions you will face are very personal. There is no single "right" or "best" option. What's right for one person won't be right for another. All choices must be respected, including the choice not to have breast reconstruction. In fact, I think the final decision is less important than having the choice.

The top priority is always to treat or prevent cancer—the ultimate goal is to achieve a cure. However, treatment decisions early on in the process can significantly impact the final results that you'll live with for the rest of your life. It is crucial to understand the long-term implications of all the decisions you and your medical team make.

If you are considering reconstruction, visit with a breast reconstruction surgeon if at all possible before any breast cancer surgery is performed. It is the only way to ensure that you are truly involved in your treatment plan. You have time. This visit with a reconstruction surgeon is unlikely to delay your cancer care or affect its outcome.

Seeing a reconstruction specialist early on will also allow you to consider "immediate breast reconstruction," which is started at the same time as your mastectomy. Most women with early-stage breast cancer and those at high risk of developing cancer are candidates. Immediate reconstruction typically provides the best final cosmetic results, minimizes scarring, and allows you to avoid the experience of living without a breast. If you are not a candidate, knowing your options for "delayed reconstruction" once your breast cancer treatment is completed can be a huge source of relief. Regardless of whether the reconstruction is immediate or delayed, most patients need more than one procedure to complete the entire reconstructive process and achieve the best results.

Today, breast cancer patients and those at high risk have many reconstructive options, including new generation breast implants and "natural" techniques like flaps and fat grafting that use a patient's own tissue. Microsurgery, an intricate, specialized type of plastic surgery, has completely revolutionized the field of breast reconstruction. Mastectomy techniques have evolved in parallel with reconstruction; skin-sparing mastectomy, and in particular nipple-sparing mastectomy, have also helped to revolutionize cosmetic outcomes after reconstruction without compromising cancer care. These advancements are likely a huge contributing factor to many women continuing to choose mastectomy and reconstruction over breast conservation (lumpectomy followed by radiation), despite the fact that studies comparing breast conservation with mastectomy show equal survival rates.

Appropriate expectations are as important in ensuring good results and patient satisfaction as your team's expertise. Breast conservation preserves as much of the patient's breast as possible and is therefore presented to patients as a means of preserving their body's physical wholeness. However, in many instances, removal of part of the breast and subsequent radiation therapy lead to a much poorer cosmetic result than anticipated, particularly in terms of breast contour and symmetry. Though low, breast cancer recurrence rates after breast conservation are also higher than with mastectomy.

Fully discussing breast reconstruction options with your surgeon can be time intensive and emotionally charged. Breast cancer patients have to deal not only with their diagnosis but also with a myriad of implications affecting their sense of mortality, body image, relationships, work, family, and social life. Women at high risk of breast cancer deal with these same issues while deciding how to reduce their chance of developing breast cancer.

Considering your surgical options can also be an exceptionally frustrating process. The most common sources of frustration are lack of appropriate, timely information and not feeling properly involved in decision making when it comes to the treatment plan. Studies have shown that patients who are involved in their treatment decision process have better outcomes. A study evaluating quality of online information to support patient decision making in breast cancer surgery found that while the information is plentiful, most of it does "a poor job providing women with essential information necessary to actively participate in decision making for breast cancer surgery."*

This newest edition of *The Breast Reconstruction Guidebook* will arm you with the latest information on *all* of your mastectomy and post-mastectomy options. Most importantly, it will empower you to take an active role in the shared decision-making process with your surgical team, regardless of your treatment choices. This in turn will make you more comfortable with your treatment plan, and you will feel more prepared for what lies ahead.

I wish you all the best.

---

*Bruce JG, Tucholka JL, Steffens NM, et al. "Quality of online information to support patient decision-making in breast cancer surgery." *Journal of Surgical Oncology* 112, no. 6 (2015): 575–80.

Acknowledgments

Sincere thanks to the many patients, physicians, reviewers, and others who continue to support this book as a resource for women who are looking for information and answers.

THE BREAST RECONSTRUCTION GUIDEBOOK

Introduction

If you're facing mastectomy to treat or prevent breast cancer, you have a lot of decisions before you. Will you keep a flat chest after surgery, wear temporary breast prostheses, or have your breasts reconstructed? If you do want to have breast reconstruction, is your priority to have the shortest procedure with the quickest recovery or to pursue a method that will give you the most natural breasts possible? Does keeping your own nipples and areolae appeal to you? Do you have quite a bit of excess fat that you'd like to be rid of in the process?

Plastic surgeons have been recreating breasts for decades. Technological innovation and surgical improvements in the 15 years since *The Breast Reconstruction Guidebook* was first published now make reconstructive results with breast implants or your own tissue better than ever. If you're interested in breast implants, you might choose cohesive silicone gel "gummy bears" that retain their shape and feel more like breast tissue. If you'd like to avoid the traditional method of tissue expansion that creates a space to hold your implant, you might be a candidate for nipple-sparing mastectomy with a direct-to-implant procedure, which completes in a single visit to the operating room what reconstruction with tissue expanders takes months to accomplish. (Solid data show that nipple-sparing mastectomy, considered to be unwise just a few years ago, is safe for most women, even many who are treated for breast cancer.) If your reconstruction is done with tissue expanders, perhaps you'll prefer to control the speed of your expansion at home, avoiding routine office visits and shortening the overall reconstruction process.

"Flaps" of your own excess fat can also be sculpted into new breasts. Plastic surgeons continue to push the reconstructive envelope, developing better flap techniques and procedures that provide more predictable results and shorten recovery. Some tissue flaps use muscle along with skin and fat to rebuild the breast, but other more sophisticated options spare the muscle, preserving function and making for less intense recovery. These micro-surgical tissue flaps, including DIEP (deep inferior epigastric perforator), GAP (gluteal artery perforator), TUG (transverse upper gracilis), and others, are no longer considered weird or experimental, and options for rebuilding your breasts with excess fat from your abdomen, back, buttocks, thighs, or hips are numerous. And flap reconstruction comes with a bonus: new breasts *and* a slimmer donor area. Methods of nipple reconstruction have also improved. Or like a growing number of women, you may prefer to have three-dimensional nipples tattooed onto your reconstructed breast, giving a lifelike illusion of having nipples where there aren't any.

One of the most exciting reconstructive innovations is fat grafting—liposuctioning your own excess fat and carefully injecting small amounts into your reconstructed breast. Although fat grafting has been used for many years, recent improvements make it far more practical and success-ful, ensuring that more fat stays in the breast. Adding fat to the new breast can refine shape, increase volume, and improve contour with minimal downtime, making a good reconstruction even better. Perhaps the most important change is the increasing number of plastic surgeons who now routinely offer breast reconstruction, translating to more accessible expe-rience, skill, and choice.

One thing that hasn't changed in 15 years is that women who consider breast reconstruction share a common dilemma: "What is the best option for me?" Because no single procedure is right for all women, the wisest ap-proach is to first carefully consider the alternatives; consult with two or three experienced, skilled surgeons; and then determine which reconstruc-tive method, if any, matches your personal preferences and priorities. For-tunately, mastectomy and reconstruction are no longer one-size-fits-all. You have options, but that also means you need to make decisions. You may not be a candidate for all procedures. If you've undergone radiation for breast cancer, for example, that poses some reconstructive limitations. Some choices may not be available in your area or within your health insur-ance network. Others may not interest you, because of the investment in time or recovery. With you in the driver's seat, you're less likely to have regrets about how your reconstruction is done, and you'll know what to expect in the hospital and at home during recovery.

Like its preceding versions, this edition of *The Breast Reconstruction Guidebook* was written to answer your questions, demystify confusing terms and concepts, and help you go from confused to confident. The text is deliberately objective. It doesn't favor or recommend one procedure or another, because that's up to you to decide.

What's most important, particularly if you're feeling that you'll never be the same, is that after mastectomy, you can have symmetrical, soft, rounded breasts. They won't feel the same as your natural breasts, but many women find that their new breasts look as good or better. Reconstruction isn't perfect, and it isn't always easy. It can't undo everything mastectomy takes away or replace lost sensation or the ability to breastfeed. But it can restore your post-mastectomy profile and profoundly affect your self-image and peace of mind, so that you can get on with your life, while you wear all the clothes you wore before your mastectomy and look natural again without your clothes.

As someone who has twice confronted breast cancer and twice had reconstruction, I understand just how you feel. I know firsthand that sorting through the various reconstructive options can be a confusing, time-intensive, and frustrating experience. By the time you've read through this book, you'll feel more confident in your choices and understanding of mastectomy and reconstruction. You may decide to go ahead with reconstruction. You may not. Either way, you'll know what to expect. And even if you decide that reconstruction is not for you, after reading through different parts of the book, you'll have a good understanding of breast cancer, mastectomy without reconstruction, and what to expect from your surgery and recovery.

How will the next 15 years change mastectomy and breast reconstruction? I hope that science is driving us toward a time when mastectomy will be archaic, and this book will be obsolete. But discovery isn't easy, and the development process isn't quick. Sooner or later, scientists will discover how to repair defective genes that cause disease. Women diagnosed with breast cancer may undergo gene therapy without needing chemotherapy or radiation. We'll move breast cancer to the list of diseases we no longer need to fear, and mastectomy will no longer be needed. Until then, reconstruction is our best antidote for replacing lost breasts.

PART ONE ○ DECISION: MASTECTOMY

CHAPTER ONE

Why Mastectomy?

This is something that no one would truly understand unless they've been there. —MARIA

As women, our breasts feed our babies, provide pleasure, and define much of our physical profile. It's heartbreaking to lose a part of us that is so uniquely feminine, and it's natural to have concerns about losing one or both breasts: Will mastectomy eliminate our cancer? How will we look afterward, when we are clothed, and when we are not? Will we ever feel normal again? In most situations, removing breast tissue (often combined with other treatment) does eliminate breast cancer. Afterward, talented plastic surgeons using sophisticated techniques can restore breast volume and shape with manufactured implants or your own tissue.

Although early Egyptians are generally credited with the initial written description of breast cancer, Greek physicians in AD 180 may have been the first to recommend surgery to remove a breast tumor.[1] By the 1700s, surgery was considered to be the most appropriate breast cancer treatment. A letter in 1811 written by English novelist Fanny Burney to her sister describing how her breast was removed by one of Napoleon's surgeons is believed to be the first documented evidence of mastectomy. Fortified with just a single wine cordial, Burney's operation was successful, and she lived for another 29 years. Seventy years later, renowned surgeon William Halsted introduced the *radical mastectomy*, with two benefits his predecessors didn't have: anesthesia and sterilized surgical instruments. At the time, the biology of breast cancer wasn't understood sufficiently to address individual condition and tumor size or to provide treatment choices. Breast cancer was recognized as a local disease best treated by removing the entire breast, the chest wall muscles, and all underarm lymph nodes, leaving women with a flat or concave chest, arm weakness, and in some cases, lifelong lingering pain. Absent other effective, more conservative methods, Halsted's procedure became standard treatment for most women diagnosed with breast cancer, and although it was disfiguring, it saved many women's lives. In the late 1970s, surgeons discovered that, for most women, removing only the tumor and breast tissue was as effective and far less debilitating.

Surgeons are still key players in almost all breast cancer diagnoses, but they are now participants in multidisciplinary medical teams that assess and coordinate each patient's treatment. Despite encouraging advances that find more breast cancers at an early stage when they're easier to treat, we still haven't cracked the cancer code. While we're beginning to understand the nature of certain breast cancers, we don't yet know how to prevent or cure all of them. We've learned that breast cancer is not one but many different diseases that must be approached in different ways. That realization has helped experts replace the one-size-fits-all treatment approach with treatment choices that are more focused, more personalized, and more successful.

In the United States, breast cancer is the second-most commonly diagnosed cancer in women (after skin cancer) and the second highest cause of cancer death (after lung cancer). Although most women survive treatment, annually 1 in 8 are diagnosed, and more than 40,000 lose their lives to this disease.[2] Many more, even those with early-stage disease, lose their breasts because of this dreaded disease or in an effort to prevent it: more than 100,000 mastectomies are performed each year in the United States.

Inside the Breast

Breasts are designed to make milk. Positioned over the *pectoralis major* and *pectoralis minor* chest muscles, milk-producing *lobules* are connected to thin *ducts* that deliver milk to the nipple. Most breast cancers begin in the ducts. The remainder of the breast is primarily fatty tissue (figure 1.1). Breasts contain no muscle—that's why no amount of exercise makes them bigger. In our twenties and thirties, our breasts have more dense glandular tissue than fat. This tissue makes the youthful breast firm. It's also the reason *mammograms* aren't routinely recommended for women under age 40, because they cannot always find abnormalities in dense tissue, and tend to produce more false positive results, meaning that additional testing or a biopsy shows that the suspicious area is not cancer. *Magnetic resonance imaging (MRI)* is more sensitive and can better distinguish suspicious areas in dense tissue; it finds more abnormalities, both harmless and harmful. As we age—particularly after menopause—our breast volume consists more of fat, and our once-firm breasts begin to sag. Though not usually welcomed or desired, aging breast tissue bodes well for early detection, because on a mammogram, fat stands out in contrast to abnormalities.

We all dread the "C" word. But what, exactly, is cancer? It occurs when environmental, lifestyle, or hereditary factors cause cells—in this case, breast cells—to mutate and grow uncontrollably until they form *malignant* (cancerous) tumors. The tumors continue to develop, usually without symptoms, until they form a spot that shows up on a mammogram or a lump that can be felt.

Breast cancer is a term that encompasses different types of malignancies in the breast. *Non-invasive breast cancers* remain in situ, or "in place," within the confines of the lobules or ducts where they begin. *Ductal carcinoma in situ (DCIS)* is disease that is contained within the ducts. Too small to be felt, it's the earliest form of breast cancer (stage 0), and the most common non-invasive type of the disease. DCIS isn't life

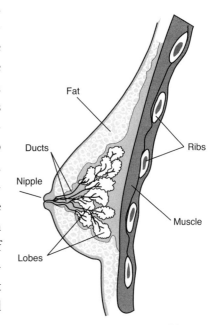

FIGURE 1.1. The breast is made of fatty tissue, lobes, and ducts surrounded by skin.

threatening and treatment is successful in virtually all cases, but it does increase the chance for developing *invasive* breast cancer, which is more worrisome, because it can spread beyond the breast to other parts of the body where it is more difficult to treat. While high-grade, fast-growing DCIS tumors may be more likely to mutate into invasive cancer, research suggests that some slow-growing DCIS tumors do not affect survival, and that close surveillance rather than treatment may be appropriate, in the same way early-stage prostate cancer is now viewed. Until experts can reliably predict which DCIS cases are likely to become invasive, surgery with or without radiation and/or hormonal therapy is still recommended.

Invasive or *infiltrating ductal carcinoma* (*IDC*) is the most common breast cancer. Usually found in women older than age 55, it begins in the ducts and spreads to the breast tissue. *Invasive lobular carcinoma* begins in the lobules. Less common types of breast cancer can develop in the breast skin, nipple, or *areola* (the darker skin around the nipple). The American Cancer Society (www.cancer.org) has detailed information about different types of breast cancer and how they are treated.

Surgical Treatments

A breast *biopsy*—a small sample of tissue or cells that is removed surgically or with a special needle—helps to determine whether cancer is present. Most biopsies prove to be *benign* (non-cancerous). When a biopsy reveals cancerous cells, your medical team will design the best course of treatment based on the type of cancer, how far it has progressed, and other factors. Treatment may include *chemotherapy* or *radiation therapy* to destroy cancer cells, medication to block the hormones that some tumors need to grow, or targeted therapy that restricts or blocks proteins or other substances that certain cancers need to thrive.

No matter what the treatment plan, some type of surgery is always involved when breast cancer is diagnosed. But, thankfully, the days of routine radical mastectomy are behind us. We live in an age of patient participation, and, when prudent, procedures that save most of the breast are often effective. Women with a single, small tumor that hasn't spread beyond the breast can choose breast-conserving *lumpectomy*: removal of just the tumor and a margin of surrounding tissue (which must be clear of cancer cells), usually followed by radiation treatments, which cut the risk of recurrence in half and improves survival.[3] When a larger tumor is involved, a *quadrantectomy*, which removes about a quarter of the breast, may be appropriate. When lumpectomy or quadrantectomy can't eliminate cancer, treatment usually involves breast removal. *Unilateral* mastectomy removes one breast; *bilateral,* or double, mastectomy removes both breasts (figure 1.2).

Depending on your diagnosis, you may have a choice between lumpectomy with radiation or mastectomy. Mastectomy is usually recommended when:

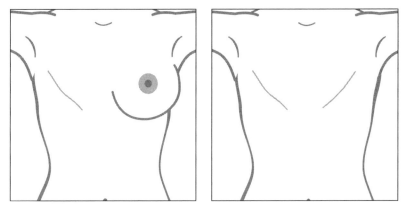

FIGURE 1.2. A unilateral mastectomy leaves one side of the chest flat (*left*). Both sides are flat after a bilateral mastectomy (*right*).

- cancer is found in multiple areas of your breast
- lumpectomy can't remove all of your cancer
- removing your tumor would eliminate a large portion of your breast
- you've had prior radiation to your breast or chest
- you have rheumatoid arthritis, lupus, or another health condition that precludes having radiation
- you're pregnant (because radiation can harm the fetus, mastectomy is usually recommended during the first trimester; during the second and third trimesters, most women, depending on the nature of their tumors, have the choice of mastectomy or lumpectomy with radiation that is delayed until after delivery)
- you have a high risk for breast cancer due to a genetic mutation, a strong family history, or a diagnosis of lobular carcinoma in situ

The type of mastectomy you have depends on the nature of your breast cancer. A *total* mastectomy removes the entire breast tissue and may include the nipple and areola. This surgery is commonly used to treat DCIS in multiple areas of the breast or when the cancerous area extends beyond the edges of the biopsy. It is also used prophylactically in women who have an inherited predisposition to breast cancer. A *modified radical mastectomy* is similar but also removes some or all underarm *lymph nodes* (part of the body's immune system that filters bacteria and cellular waste materials) and the lining over the chest muscle. The Halsted radical mastectomy is uncommon, unless advanced tumors are found in the chest muscle.

> *There are absolutely no words to describe the stress and anxiety that un-*
> *expectedly creeps up about having mastectomy. I wish I could tell some-*
> *one, "This is how I feel," but I can't. Anything I say about it, any way*
> *I describe it, is inadequate. I love and appreciate each and every person*
> *who supports me and cares about me more than anyone will ever know.*
> *But this is something that no one would truly understand unless they've*
> *been there.*   —Maria

Finding malignant cells in the underarm lymph nodes (figure 1.3) in-dicates that cancer has spread beyond the breast and is capable of *metasta-sis* (spread) to other parts of the body. If you have invasive breast cancer, any underarm lymph nodes on the same side as the breast tumor that look or feel enlarged or unusual will be removed during your lumpectomy or mastectomy. If your cancer was identified at an early stage and your nodes appear normal, your surgeon will do a *sentinel lymph node biopsy* (*SLNB*). This is also called *sentinel lymph node dissection* or *sentinel lymph node mapping*. Cancer cells that spread beyond the breast initially travel to the sentinel node, the one that is closest to the tumor, so typically, when early-stage cancer is found, only this node is removed and examined. Sometimes, one or two adjacent nodes are removed as well. A sentinel node that is clear of cancer cells is great news—the rest of your lymph nodes are also presumed to be clear. Guidelines from the American Soci-ety of Clinical Oncology define SLNB as appropriate for women with early-stage breast cancer who:

- have DCIS that is treated with mastectomy
- have operable, multicentric tumors (tumors that form separately)
- have previously had breast cancer surgery or axillary lymph node surgery
- had chemotherapy or other preoperative systemic treatment

SLNB is not appropriate for women who are pregnant, have inflammatory breast cancer, have lumpectomy to treat DCIS, or have tumors that are

5 cm or larger or have spread extensively in the breast or to nearby lymph nodes.[4]

When cancer cells are found in the sentinel node, an *axillary lymph node dissection (ALND)* will remove some or all of your underarm lymph nodes to determine whether cancer has invaded and chemotherapy or other systemic treatment is needed. No additional nodes need to be removed if the sentinel node is clear of cancer cells, or only one or two sentinel nodes are positive for cancer cells and you're planning to have radiation therapy after lumpectomy. ALND is recommended, however, if cancer cells are found in your sentinel node and you plan to have a mastectomy.

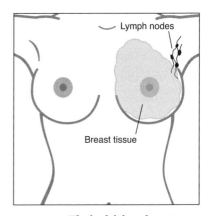

FIGURE 1.3. The body's lymph system includes small underarm nodes that filter impurities from the body.

While ALND is a critical diagnostic step, it can impair the lymph system's ability to adequately filter body fluids, which may then collect in the arm, causing mild to severe *lymphedema*, a lifelong condition characterized by chronic swelling and numbness that can occur months or even years after nodes are removed. Up to 30 percent of women who have axillary node dissection develop lymphedema, compared with about 3 percent who have a less invasive sentinel node procedure.[5] Radiating the lymph nodes also increases the risk for lymphedema; however, some research involving patients with positive sentinel nodes shows that radiating the axillary lymph nodes is as effective as removing them and lowers the risk of lymphedema.[6] More study is needed, and axillary dissection might still be advisable for women whose nodes are palpable or contain breast cancer cells.

Male Mastectomy

All women are at risk for breast cancer, but the threat extends to men as well, and it can be just as serious. The estimated lifetime risk for men is quite low, about 1 in 1,000 compared to 1 in 8 women. Nevertheless, male breast cancer does occur. It's more common in men over the age of 60, although men of any age can be diagnosed. The risk is greater for men with an inherited predisposition to breast cancer (chapter 5).

Because men have far less breast tissue than women, a man's tumor tends to involve a greater portion of the breast than the same size tumor in a woman. Lumpectomy followed by radiation may be an option when the tumor is present only in the nipple, but generally, modified radical mastectomy is recommended. The breast tissue, nipple, and areola are removed along with some axillary lymph nodes. Radiation, chemotherapy, hormonal therapy, and/or targeted therapy may also be recommended.

Men don't typically need reconstruction after mastectomy, because the amount of tissue removed isn't usually enough to disfigure the breast; any cosmetic irregularities can usually be remedied with small fat grafts (chapter 10). Nipple reconstruction and/or a tattoo that simulates the nipple and areola are also options.

Do You Really Need a Mastectomy?

Depending on the nature of your cancer, you may have a choice between lumpectomy with radiation or mastectomy. Given the option to save your breast, why would you choose to remove it instead? Personal reasons may compel you to opt for mastectomy: you may live too far from a treatment facility, you may be unable to accommodate the schedule of radiation appointments, or you might simply prefer to avoid the potential side effects of radiation, including potentially less-than-satisfactory results from breast reconstruction. The likelihood of a recurrence is slightly higher after lumpectomy and radiation than mastectomy. Mastectomy would be necessary if your cancer returns, because it isn't safe to radiate the same breast more than once. If you have an unusually high risk of developing a recurrence or another new tumor, you may feel that removing your breast will give you greater peace of mind.

Compared to most other developed nations, the rate of mastectomy is higher in the United States, especially among younger women with non-invasive disease, smaller tumors, and node-negative disease—all indications that the cancers are less likely to spread beyond the initial tumor.[7] Widespread media coverage of celebrity mastectomies is likely one reason for the increase. Where you live in the United States may also make a difference: lumpectomy is more common in the Northeast and Pacific West, while mastectomy occurs more often in the South and parts of the Midwest.[8]

Physicians are more likely to recommend breast-conserving lumpectomy in metropolitan areas and locations where radiation facilities are plentiful. Your surgeon's age and medical training may also influence his or her treatment recommendation. Despite statistics showing that lumpectomy with radiation is as effective as mastectomy, patients often prefer mastectomy because they worry about their cancer returning, because of the side effects of radiation, or because preoperative screening shows additional areas of concern in the breast. Preventive bilateral mastectomy may also be recommended if you are genetically predisposed to breast cancer (more on this in chapter 5).

Contralateral mastectomy. Diagnosed with cancer in one breast, it's natural to fear a future diagnosis in the opposite breast. That's likely the most common reason why many women who face unilateral mastectomy choose to remove their healthy breast as well. This *contralateral prophylactic mastectomy (CPM)* isn't recommended for most breast cancer patients because it doesn't improve survival, and fewer than 10 percent of women who have lumpectomy and radiation or unilateral mastectomy develop cancer in the opposite breast.[9]

Despite the lack of benefit for most women, the rate of CPM tripled over a decade, from about 4 percent in 2002 to about 13 percent in 2012, and nearly doubled in men between 2004 and 2011.[10] So why remove a perfectly healthy breast and have additional surgery you don't need? Mostly, it appears that women diagnosed with breast cancer in one breast choose CPM to gain peace of mind but they overestimate their risk for cancer in the opposite breast. Increasing use of pre-mastectomy MRIs, which sometimes show early-stage abnormalities in the opposite breast (and can produce false positive results) probably also play a role. Women who have pre-mastectomy MRIs choose contralateral mastectomy twice as often as those who don't.[11] Reconstruction may also be a deciding factor; better symmetry, particularly for women with large, drooping breasts, is more likely when both breasts are removed and reconstructed at the same time.

Contralateral mastectomy is recommended for a small percentage of women, including those with a high risk of recurrence, a genetic mutation that increases breast cancer risk, or a family history of breast or ovarian cancer. For some women, particularly those who would like to retain

TABLE 1.1. Comparing lumpectomy and mastectomy

Lumpectomy	Mastectomy
Minimal surgery	More extensive surgery
May affect appearance of your breast	Removes your breast
Outpatient procedure	Usually requires overnight hospital stay
Requires follow-up radiation treatments	May require follow-up radiation treatments
Continued mammograms advised	Mammograms no longer needed*
Sensation retained	Sensation reduced or eliminated
Reconstruction not usually needed	Reconstruction is always an option
Slightly higher chance of recurrence	Same survival rate as lumpectomy and radiation

*After unilateral mastectomy, routine mammograms of your healthy breast are still recommended.

at least one breast with normal sensation, removing their remaining, healthy breast may be unacceptable. A bilateral mastectomy means a longer operation and additional opportunity for infection and other post-op complications. If you're facing unilateral mastectomy, having an accurate perception of your risk and understanding your options to reduce recurrence will help you decide whether you should remove your other breast as well.

If you have a choice of lumpectomy or mastectomy, you may be conflicted by the emotional and intellectual factors involved in the decision. Understandably, you'll be anxious to get rid of the source of your cancer—your breasts—and feel safer when you do. It's a difficult decision that is best made by weighing all the advantages and disadvantages of each option. Only you can make that decision. You may decide that mastectomy is your best option, but before you do, give yourself time to understand all the facts and consider all your options (table 1.1). Unless you have a very aggressive cancer, taking two or three weeks to get a second opinion will be well worth your time. You have nothing to lose, and it just might save your breast. If you decide mastectomy is your best course of action, you have choices about how you'll look after your breast is removed.

CHAPTER TWO

Mastectomy without Reconstruction

*Mastectomy scars are a reminder that you've lost a breast;
they're also a reminder that you've survived.*

—MASTECTOMY PATIENT

Discussions about whether women should have breast reconstruction after mastectomy are like politics: everyone has an opinion. Wander around the Internet and you'll find vehement blogs against reconstruction, arguing why women should stay flat after mastectomy. You'll also find the polar opposite view: strongly worded positions in favor of breast reconstruction. As women, we are all different. We have different goals, varying likes and dislikes, and decidedly contrasting opinions of what is right for each of us. Some of us feel the breast reconstruction journey is worth the effort, and that is just fine. Others consider it a waste of time and effort, and that is also fine, because what is right for one isn't necessarily right for all. You might decide against reconstruction if you:

- don't want to endure additional surgery and recovery
- want the simplest and fastest recovery
- don't consider a flat chest to be a significant change from your natural breasts
- fear potential reconstructive complications or unsatisfactory results
- don't want breasts that aren't "real" and have little or no feeling
- want to try going flat before committing to reconstructive surgery
- are unsure about reconstruction at the time of your mastectomy
- have a health condition or pending treatment that precludes reconstruction
- prefer to embrace your flat chest as a way of acknowledging your post-cancer persona

What to Expect

The goal of mastectomy is always to remove as much breast tissue as possible, whether or not you have reconstruction. If you don't have reconstruction at the time of your mastectomy, a broad elliptical incision is made across your breast, removing the nipple and areola and any previous biopsy scars. The breast tissue, tumor, and most of the skin are removed. The edges of skin on either side of the incision are pulled together and closed around a surgical drain, which remains in place for a few days to drain fluids away from your chest while you heal (more on drains in chapter 15).

Surgery to perform a unilateral mastectomy lasts an hour or so, while the entire bilateral process takes about two to three hours, depending on the nature of your mastectomy. Patients usually spend at least one night in the hospital, although some go home the same day. You'll be up and walking around the next day; however, you'll need extra rest for several days. A nurse will demonstrate gentle (but important) movements to prevent stiffness in your shoulder and arm. Performing these exercises daily will gradually restore full range of motion and strength in your chest, shoulders, and arm. While you'll become a bit stronger each day, you may need four to six weeks before you're able to resume all of your normal routine.

Unless complications occur, you may be surprised to feel little or no pain after mastectomy, because nerves are severed when tissue is removed. Your chest will be numb and may feel heavy, and you may feel a pulling sensation under your arm; this improves as your chest heals. Prescribed medication will control any discomfort in the first few days after your surgery, and then you can use over-the-counter medication as you need it. Ideally, your breast surgeon will try to leave your chest surface as smooth as possible. Your chest will be flat or slightly concave. Initially, your incision will be red and prominent. It fades noticeably after several months but remains across your chest, even if you have reconstruction later on. As more than one patient has said, mastectomy scars are a reminder that you've lost a breast; they're also a reminder that you've survived. Three informative sources about mastectomy without reconstruction are Breast-Free (www.breastfree.org), Flat & Fabulous (www.flatandfabulous.org), and BreastHealing.com (www.breasthealing.com).

Having a BRCA1 mutation, my risk reduction plan included preventative mastectomies without reconstruction. As a physician and a caregiver for a cancer patient, I wanted to quickly get back to my life. I felt lucky that my lifestyle, personality, and relationships weren't focused on my breasts, and I didn't want to bother with mastectomy bras and prostheses. With no reconstruction to worry about, I had only minor issues with healing, which weren't at all traumatic. But I worried about what people would think about my choice, and how I would cope with prominent scars; they run unevenly across my chest with an inch gap in-between, which isn't the ideal cosmetic appearance. After a year, they faded to my natural skin color. Three years later, I'm proud and pleased to have acted so quickly and adapted so well to this big challenge and major surgery. I've moved forward with my life, and I never worry about how my activities will affect my chest. I'm confident in my ability to do a self-exam of my chest and find any future cancer. My scars sometimes attract my attention when I look in the mirror—often I just see me. And no one has ever commented about noticing that I go flat. I wouldn't have done anything differently. —Margaret*

I had an epiphany when I woke up after my mastectomy: I thought I would lose my sex appeal and femininity, but that didn't happen. I spent many years with a knock-out curvaceous body, now I'm okay with the new me and I've never regretted my decision. I found my spirit, my beauty, my confidence . . . myself. I've never worn my breast forms. I go flat and I'm not embarrassed. I look great and I'm still turning heads; most people don't even know I have no breasts. A surprising benefit to having no breasts is that when I hug my husband, we are chest to chest, skin to skin—closer than we ever were before when my breasts were "in the way." It's a nice feeling. —Sangria*

The Prosthesis Alternative

After mastectomy, you may prefer a flat chest, or you may like to wear a *prosthesis*, a breast-shaped form worn under your clothes. Tucked into pockets of specially made bras, lingerie, and swimsuits, prostheses restore shape and profile. (Partial prostheses are also available to fill out post-lumpectomy indentations in the top, bottom, or side of your breast.) You can also buy sew-in pockets to modify bras to hold prostheses. If you're handy with a needle and thread, you can alter just about any bra yourself (search the Internet for "sew-in mastectomy pockets"). Some prostheses adhere to your chest and can be worn without a bra—try one before you buy several, just in case the adhesive irritates your skin.

If both of your breasts are removed, your new "breast" size is limited only by the prostheses you choose. Unilateral mastectomy presents a more practical problem. Because one breast is missing, you may feel unbalanced or lopsided and find it difficult to fit into clothes. When you're dressed, one side of your chest will be flat; if you wear a bra, one cup will be empty. You can balance your remaining breast and regain symmetry with a weighted prosthesis that will provide balance and help you to maintain proper posture. (It's not necessary to wear a weighted prosthesis after bilateral mastectomy.) If you're undecided about reconstruction or you need to delay it until you've completed your post-mastectomy treatment, a prosthesis can serve as a temporary breast during the in-between interval.

If you contact Reach to Recovery (www.cancer.org) several weeks before your mastectomy, a volunteer will bring a lightweight starter prosthesis and a mastectomy camisole or bra to the hospital and show you how to use them. When your scar heals sufficiently—generally in about four to six weeks—your surgeon will write a prescription for mastectomy bras and more balanced, better-designed prostheses. Be sure to get a prescription; otherwise, your insurance may not cover the cost. It's a good idea to be measured by a board-certified fitter for your first prosthesis to ensure it fits properly on your chest and isn't too light or too heavy. Try on different styles to see which ones look and feel the best.

Types of prostheses. Prostheses are available in different shapes (figure 2.1), skin tones, and materials and vary in cost. Inexpensive cotton, foam, and fiberfill prostheses are comfortable and fill a bra; however, they provide the least shape. Soft gel prostheses are lighter and feel better. Silicone breast forms feel and look the most natural—they're also the most expensive—and most closely mimic the weight of a natural breast (the silicone used is different than the material used in breast implants). You can buy them with or without nipples; you can also buy stick-on nipples. Silicone prostheses are heavier than cotton, foam, or gel and can be uncomfortably hot in the summer or when a menopausal hot flash occurs. Lightweight

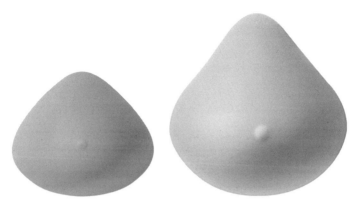

FIGURE 2.1. A triangular prosthesis fills in missing tissue at the sides and top of the breast (*left*). A teardrop prosthesis gives extra fullness at the bottom (*right*). Photos courtesy of Amoena USA Corporation.

silicone prostheses are also available. Very light breast forms made of thousands of plastic microbeads and covered with soft fabric are another alternative; they're like beanbags with tiny beads that mold to your body. Visit the Breastfree website or Knitted Knockers (www.knittedknockers.org) for details about making your own soft breast forms.

Where to shop. Nordstrom, Sears, Lands' End, and JCPenney sell mastectomy garments and prostheses online, from catalogs, and in their store lingerie departments. Post-mastectomy boutiques are often listed online or in the phone directory under "Mastectomy Forms and Supplies" or "Prosthetics." The American Cancer Society (ACS) offers a good selection of reasonably priced prostheses and mastectomy products in its TLC catalog (www.tlcdirect.org). You'll also find a wide selection online (try www.amoena.com, www.mastectomyshop.com, and www.nearlyme.org). If you would like to explore the possibility of a prosthesis made to your exact specifications, search online for "custom breast prosthesis." It's more expensive and may not be fully covered by insurance.

Tips for buying prostheses:

- Let a qualified fitter help you find the right size.
- Take someone with you for a second opinion about how you look wearing different prostheses.

- After unilateral mastectomy, it's important to match the weight and size of your remaining breast.
- Consider prostheses of different weights and fabrics for different activities or occasions.
- If you like to swim, choose a prosthesis that won't be damaged by salt water or chlorine.

Paying for Mastectomy and Prostheses

Although most insurers cover overnight hospital stays for mastectomy, and several state laws protect your right to stay in the hospital for at least 24 or 48 hours after your surgery, some insurance companies still require "drive-through" mastectomies, providing hospital coverage only for 24 hours. Since 1996, the insurance lobby has effectively squashed several attempts to pass federal legislation that would mandate longer hospital stays after mastectomy, if needed. With ongoing concerns about hospital-acquired infections, particularly after surgery, it's advantageous to go home as soon as it's prudent for you to do so. Most women are able to go home the same or next day, but if you need an extra day or two (as determined by you and your physician), you should surely have it. Check with your health insurer to determine your coverage, and confer with your state health department to be clear about your rights.

The *Women's Health and Cancer Rights Act (WHCRA)* of 1998 requires insurance companies who pay for mastectomy to also cover prostheses. Most carriers base their coverage on Medicare guidelines. With a doctor's prescription, coverage typically includes one foam prosthesis breast (two after bilateral mastectomy) every six months and one silicone prosthesis every two years (two after bilateral mastectomy). Medicare coverage also includes four to six mastectomy bras annually, or more if your doctor says they are medically necessary—if you have additional surgery or lose or gain weight, for example. These guidelines sometimes change, so it's a good idea to check with your insurance company to see what your coverage allows. Many retailers will bill your insurance company directly after you pay a small co-payment. Other vendors may require full payment at the time of purchase; you can then request reimbursement from your insurance company. (Medicare requires a reimbursement claim directly from the supplying vendor; the reimbursement is then forwarded directly to you.)

If you don't have insurance and can't afford a prosthesis, contact your local and state cancer organizations or the following sources to explore financial assistance or the possibility of prostheses at no charge:

The American Cancer Society (www.cancer.org)
CancerCare's Linking Arms Program (www.cancercare.org)
Patient Advocate Foundation (www.copays.org)

Chapter 19 deals with insurance coverage for breast reconstruction.

CHAPTER THREE

Breast Reconstruction Basics

At 31, I just couldn't deal with having no breasts. If I had to have a mastectomy, I wanted to restore my breasts as closely as possible, and that meant reconstruction. —RILEY

Until we know how to prevent cancer, outsmart it with cellular repair, or develop treatments that make mastectomy obsolete, reconstruction is our best antidote to breast loss. Surgical reconstruction repairs cosmetic and functional defects caused by injury, trauma, or disease. Talented *plastic surgeons* rebuild facial features, repair severe burns and lacerations, and improve birth defects. They can also create breasts after mastectomy, complete with nipple and areola. Breast reconstruction is more complex and requires more surgical skill than *breast augmentation*, which uses implants or fat to increase the size of healthy breasts.

The goal of breast reconstruction used to be to restore a woman's shape when she was dressed, but the bar is now much higher: to create soft, gently sloped breasts that look natural, when you're clothed and when you're not. This is what good reconstruction does—although some results are better than others, depending on your surgeon, the procedure you choose, and your own physical makeup. You can search the Internet for "before and after breast reconstruction" to see examples of various surgeons' work. The images you find may represent only each surgeon's best results, but they'll give you an idea of what is possible and how results vary.

Breast reconstruction doesn't cause cancer, affect recurrence, or hide cancer if it recurs. While reconstruction is imperfect—it can't remove mastectomy scars, restore sensation, or reestablish your ability to breast-feed—it can soften the harshness of mastectomy and restore your feeling of physical wholeness. (It can also help if you were born with Poland's syndrome, a condition characterized by little or no breast tissue; sometimes the chest muscle is also missing or highly underdeveloped—it's like being born with a radical mastectomy.) In the right surgeon's hands, reconstructed breasts are much more than the sum of their parts. They're works of art customized to your physique and preference. Small, large, round, high, droopy—we all have different breast shapes and sizes. Good reconstruction can recreate and often improve the look of natural breasts. Because bilateral reconstruction starts with a "clean slate," some women find that their reconstructed breasts are more symmetrical, with better shape and fewer cosmetic imperfections than their natural breasts. With your breast volume and symmetry restored, you can wear the same clothes you wore before mastectomy, including lingerie, T-shirts, and bathing suits, without special bras or prostheses.

Sorting through the Options

When it comes to deciding whether to have reconstruction, there are no right or wrong answers. There are only personal decisions. For many women, deciding to have reconstruction is a no-brainer; if they're going to lose their breasts, they want to replace them. Others adamantly don't want or need reconstruction. Some women are conflicted about what they should do. No matter what you ultimately decide, you have choices after mastectomy. It pays to thoroughly research your options and know what to expect before you decide whether breast reconstruction is right for you.

At 31, I just couldn't deal with having no breasts. If I had to have mastectomy, I wanted to restore my breasts as closely as possible, and that meant reconstruction. —Riley

Because of my high inherited risk for breast cancer, having bilateral mastectomy was an easy decision and reconstruction was just part of that process. Two cousins had already been through the process—one had reconstruction, the other didn't. Both seemed happy with their outcomes, which told me there was no right way to go through this decision process; it was an individual choice. Though I had never been fond of my small ugly breasts, I thought I'd be uncomfortable without any reconstruction. Considering all the options, I joked that I was going to the "boob store" to pick out a better pair that was far less likely to kill me. Ordinarily, I would never have considered plastic surgery, so I considered this an opportunity to make me feel better about my body. I had lousy odds for breast cancer, but I was going to at least indulge myself with pretty, more proportionate breasts. I knew reconstruction was the right choice for me.   —Jennifer

The American Society of Plastic Surgeons (ASPS) reported 106,338 breast reconstruction procedures by member surgeons in 2015, compared to 62,930 in 2004. The increase can be attributed to:

- increased awareness about reconstruction
- laws that require insurance companies that cover mastectomy to also pay for reconstruction
- mastectomy techniques that preserve most breast skin, often including the nipple and areola
- improved reconstructive procedures that produce better results and shorten recovery

Women say they choose reconstruction because it:

- makes them feel whole again
- restores their confidence in their physical appearance
- gives them a sense of control they didn't have with their treatment
- isn't a constant reminder of their mastectomy, unlike a flat chest or prosthesis
- brings a sense of closure to the physical and emotional struggle of breast cancer diagnosis and treatment

The reconstruction process. Although some surgeons offer newer procedures that shorten the overall reconstruction timeline, most still use traditional methods that involve two or more operations over several months (chapters 6–12 describe reconstructive procedures). The initial surgery forms the *breast mound*—a breast without a nipple or areola—with implants, your own tissue, or a combination of both (figure 3.1). This first stage is the most complex and involves the most recovery. The second stage, performed three months or more after the initial operation, is a *revision sur-*

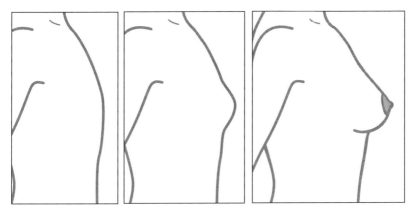

FIGURE 3.1. After mastectomy (*left*), most reconstructive procedures build the breast mound (*center*), and then later add the nipple; tattooing of the nipple and areola completes the reconstructive process (*right*).

gery to correct problems or refine aesthetics. During revision surgery, cosmetic imperfections can be improved. Fat can be added to create fullness, scars can be revised, or after *unilateral reconstruction*, your opposite healthy breast can be modified for better symmetry. Nipple reconstruction (chapter 12), if needed, is also done during revision surgery. You may go home the same day following revision surgery, or spend overnight in the hospital, depending on extent of the procedures performed.

Reconstruction with *breast implants* usually involves multiple stages over several months. Although it can also be performed in a single one-step operation without later revision surgery, temporary implants called *tissue expanders* are usually placed beneath the chest muscle and gradually inflated with saline over several weeks to stretch the skin and muscle. Then, during a later revision operation, the expander is replaced with a full-sized implant. *Tissue flaps* of your own fat, skin, and sometimes muscle can also be used to create breasts after mastectomy. Unlike most implant reconstruction, flaps form full-sized breasts during the initial operation. You go into the operating room with your natural breasts and come out with full-sized breast mounds in their place. Compared to implant reconstruction, tissue flap procedures are more complex and require greater surgical skill. Although recovery is more intense, the overall reconstruction timeline is shorter than reconstruction involving tissue expansion (table 3.1).

TABLE 3.1. Comparing implant and tissue flap procedures

Aspect of procedure	Breast implants	Tissue flaps
Surgery	Two short operations*	Longer initial operation and revision surgery
Hospital stay	1–2 days when combined with mastectomy; overnight if performed anytime after mastectomy	3–5 days whether performed with mastectomy or as a separate surgery
Recovery	Shorter	Longer
Recreating nipple	Separate procedure	Separate procedure
Scars	At mastectomy site	At mastectomy and donor sites
Modifying opposite breast (after unilateral mastectomy)	May be required to achieve symmetry	Less likely to be needed for symmetry

*Traditional procedures involving tissue expansion.

Reconstruction with implants and tissue flaps can produce good results. Research repeatedly shows that women are generally satisfied with their breast reconstruction regardless of the technique used, reporting improved breast satisfaction and psychological and sexual well-being. That doesn't mean that every woman who has breast reconstruction thinks her recreated breasts are perfect, but it does indicate that, for the most part, women who have breast reconstruction say that it has a positive impact on their post-mastectomy lives.

Timing Your Reconstruction

Your breasts can be rebuilt after your mastectomy while you're still in the operating room or anytime down the road. It's best to research reconstruction, consult with plastic surgeons, and understand different ways your breasts can be recreated before you have your mastectomy.

Immediate reconstruction. *Immediate reconstruction* is performed as soon as your mastectomy is complete, while you're still asleep on the op-

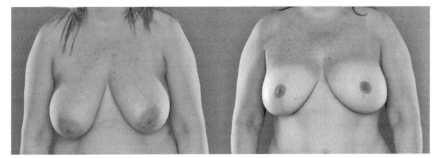

FIGURE 3.2. Immediate reconstruction replaces natural breasts (*left*) with minimal scarring and optimal cosmetic results (*right*). Images provided by Dr. Frank J. DellaCroce and The Center for Restorative Breast Surgery, LLC.

erating table. Working together, your breast surgeon and plastic surgeon will decide how your mastectomy incisions can best accommodate your reconstruction. In the operating room, the breast surgeon or *surgical oncologist* performs the mastectomy, and the plastic surgeon then steps in to do the reconstruction (figure 3.2).

Immediate reconstruction offers distinct benefits:

- Most of your breast skin is preserved.
- You may be able to keep your own nipples and areolas.
- Your mastectomy incision is less obvious and may be completely hidden.
- Your mastectomy and reconstruction are completed in a single visit to the operating room.
- You wake up from surgery with a breast mound in place, so you never experience a completely flat chest.

Delayed reconstruction. It's never too late to have your breasts recreated. A postponed or *delayed reconstruction* can be performed as a separate operation, weeks, months, or years after your mastectomy. Postponing reconstruction for up to a year after mastectomy to see whether cancer would return used to be routinely advised. Reconstruction doesn't affect recurrence, but a recurrence may affect reconstruction, and a breast implant or flap reconstruction may need to be removed to adequately treat cancer that returns. If you've been diagnosed with breast cancer, it's important to discuss with your medical team your risk of recurrence and how it might affect the timing of your reconstruction. When reconstruction

TABLE 3.2. Comparing mastectomy with and without reconstruction

Mastectomy with immediate reconstruction	Mastectomy without reconstruction
Retains most breast skin	Removes most breast skin
May retain nipple and areola	Removes nipple and areola
Two surgeries in one visit to the operating room	Single surgery
Incision is minimized and may be hidden	Incision visibly spans the chest
New breast mound after mastectomy	Flat chest after mastectomy
One or more days of hospital stay	Overnight hospital stay
Extended recovery period	Relatively short recovery period

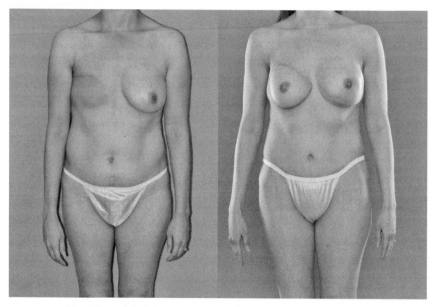

FIGURE 3.3. To perform delayed reconstruction, the mastectomy scar (*left*) is reopened to accommodate the reconstruction. The scar remains on the new breast after reconstruction (*right*) but fades in time. Images provided by Dr. Frank J. DellaCroce and The Center for Restorative Breast Surgery, LLC.

is delayed, the mastectomy procedure is the same as described in chapter 2 (table 3.2)—just enough skin is left to smoothly pull the incision closed across the chest. If you decide to reconstruct in the future, your plastic surgeon will reopen your mastectomy scar to replace your missing tissue. The scar will be prominent on your new breast, but it will fade considerably in time (figure 3.3).

It's best to delay reconstruction when:

- You're unsure about reconstruction at the time of your mastectomy.
- You want to try a prosthesis before committing to reconstructive surgery.
- You have a health condition that may add to your surgical risk or impede healing.
- Your doctor advises you to complete radiation or other cancer treatment before reconstruction.

My mastectomy was overwhelming. I just couldn't deal with reconstruction too. I changed my mind three years later when I still couldn't face myself in the mirror, and I was uncomfortable being naked around my husband. For me, delaying reconstruction was the right decision. —Copper

My oncologist suggested I wait a few months after my mastectomy to see how I felt about reconstruction. I so feared looking down and seeing only a flat, scarred chest. If I was going to lose my breast, I wanted to replace it as soon as possible. —Diana

Health Matters

Reconstruction isn't particularly dangerous, but like any surgery, complications are possible. Mastectomy and immediate reconstruction are more complex and invasive than mastectomy alone and is more likely to create post-op problems. Though it doesn't guarantee you won't have a problem or two, the more fit you are, the better you'll weather the experience, including older women who generally experience the same benefits from reconstruction as younger women. Women well into their seventies and beyond have had successful reconstruction (even though many physicians don't discuss post-mastectomy options with older women, because they assume women of a certain age aren't interested). Age doesn't automatically equate to more problems, although older women may have more health issues that may be problematic when combined with surgery. Compared to their younger counterparts, women who are age 60 or older have only slightly more post-surgical issues after implant or tissue flap reconstruction than younger women.[1] Older women, however, have significantly higher risk for *venous thromboembolism,* a blood clot that develops in a deep vein of the leg or lungs, so certain precautions, including the use of blood-thinning medications, are needed.[2]

Your doctor may advise against reconstructive surgery if your overall health is poor or you have heart or lung disease or chronic high blood pressure. Having lupus, scleroderma, rheumatoid arthritis, and other autoimmune diseases can increase the risk of poor wound healing and infection. If you're diabetic, your chances of complications are greater with tissue flap reconstruction than implant procedures, whether or not you are insulin dependent.[3]

Obesity. Obesity doesn't automatically limit your ability to have either immediate or delayed reconstruction (figure 3.4). Obese women are just

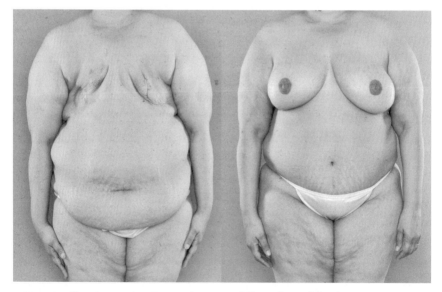

FIGURE 3.4. Breast reconstruction can be successfully performed for obese women, although they may experience more complications from surgery. Images provided by Dr. Frank J. DellaCroce and The Center for Restorative Breast Surgery, LLC.

TABLE 3.3. Body mass index (BMI) classifications

Classification of body weight	BMI score*
Normal	20–25
Overweight	25–30
Obese	Over 30
Morbidly obese[†]	40 or higher

*BMI formula: your weight in pounds $\times\, 703 \div$ (your height in inches)^2. For example, a woman who is 5′6″ and weighs 205 pounds has a BMI of 33 (205 $\times$ 703 $\div$ 4356).
[†]100 pounds or more over ideal body weight.

as likely to be satisfied with the results of their reconstruction as thinner women, but they have more post-op infections, delayed wound healing, clotting, and often require a longer hospital stay and readmission at some point.[4] The higher your body mass index (BMI), the greater your risk for complications, regardless of the reconstructive procedure you have (table 3.3). Having an experienced reconstructive surgeon, especially one who is experienced in performing procedures for obese women, can result in fewer problems and better manageability when they do occur. Flap reconstruction has a lower failure rate among heavier women, tends to provide more natural-looking breasts than implants, and provides improved body contour at the donor site. If you are very heavy, even the largest implant may not provide the adequate volume and projection you'd like, while your own fat most likely will.

Smoking. Smoking compromises your overall health. It also greatly increases the chances of postoperative complications, including excessive scarring, poor healing, and especially infection. Carbon monoxide and nicotine from tobacco products compromise healing by reducing respiratory capability and restricting blood flow to the tissues. If you smoke, you're more likely to experience *necrosis*, or tissue death, in your remaining breast skin and reconstructed breast. This means the skin or tissue dies because it doesn't get enough blood and oxygen. While this isn't optimal for implant reconstruction, it can be disastrous for breasts created with your own tissue. If you hope to have reconstruction, you'll need to stop smoking several weeks before and after your surgery—you don't want to go to the trouble of having reconstruction only to compromise the outcome and potentially lose your new breasts. The good news is that avoiding all tobacco products can reduce your odds of having problems.

Coordinating Reconstruction with Treatment

While breast reconstruction can restore your breasts and provide a tremendous psychological boost, treating your cancer is always your medical team's first priority. *Neoadjuvant* (before mastectomy) therapy generally doesn't affect the timing of reconstruction. In some cases, *adjuvant* (after mastectomy) therapy may delay it.

Reconstruction and chemotherapy. Some side effects from chemotherapy can be difficult to handle, but for women with invasive breast cancer, chemo reduces recurrence and improves survival. Fearing that potential infection or slow-healing wounds after reconstruction might delay adjuvant chemotherapy, many oncologists prefer to err on the side of caution and recommend delaying reconstruction for three to six months after chemo has been completed. This gives your body time to recover before you have an invasive reconstructive procedure, but the delay can be a disappointing turn of events, especially if you dread the thought of waking up from your mastectomy without breasts. In fact, research shows that, for most women, immediate reconstruction doesn't significantly delay chemotherapy, and when postoperative complications occur, the resulting delay in chemotherapy isn't clinically significant.[5] Implant reconstruction is less invasive than tissue flap procedures and is less likely to result in problems that might delay chemo. In most cases involving adjuvant chemo, an expander can be placed at the time of mastectomy, and chemo can be delayed for four to six weeks as the expansion process is accelerated and completed. If your oncologist recommends immediate chemotherapy, your expander can be inflated during your treatment. If you don't feel up to the expansion process (described in chapter 7), it can be delayed until you complete your chemo regimen. Exchanging the expander for an implant and creating a new nipple must wait until your immune system recovers, usually three to six months after your final chemo session. Your oncologist, plastic surgeon, and others on your health care team will determine the best timing for your reconstruction, depending on your treatment plan and overall health.

I was disappointed when my oncologist said I should delay reconstruction for at least a year after my mastectomy. Intellectually, I knew chemo was more important, but emotionally, I didn't want to be without breasts. I'm glad I waited, because it gave me time to think about my options. —Kandy

Reconstruction and radiation. The ideal reconstruction involves skin that hasn't been radiated, but that's a luxury not all women have. More breast cancer patients, especially those with tumors that are 4 cm or larger or with positive lymph nodes, have radiation therapy to destroy any remaining cancer cells in the breast. Radiation therapy is an effective cancer killer—high-energy radiation x-rays disrupt the DNA of cancer cells so that they're unable to reproduce. But it also permanently changes the molecular structure of remaining healthy tissue, reducing blood flow and elasticity in the skin. Radiation delivered before or after mastectomy can compromise breast shape, volume, and position, regardless of the type of reconstruction performed. A delay of six months or more after radiation is often advised so the skin can heal before having reconstruction. Long-term cosmetic outcome after radiation tends to be better with delayed reconstruction.

Asked which reconstruction has the most complications, surgeons will probably answer without hesitation: "Implant reconstruction after radiation." The combination is not the best, and results are difficult to predict. Some women have satisfactory reconstructive outcomes after radiation, but the odds of having problems, including implant replacement, are high (figure 3.5). Radiated skin can be difficult to expand, and it's more likely to develop infection, heal slowly, or break down from the pressure of the expander or implant. Slow, conservative expansion (with a tissue expander) sometimes works; frequently, it does not. Expanders and implants produce better results and fewer complications when they're placed before radiation; even then, radiation may compromise or sabotage the reconstruction. Compared with breasts rebuilt with your own living tissue, adjuvant

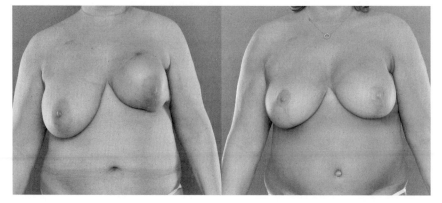

FIGURE 3.5. After radiation therapy, a breast that is reconstructed with an implant can become hard and distorted (*left*). This patient's implant was replaced with a soft tissue flap, and the opposite untreated breast was lifted for better symmetry (*right*). Images provided by Dr. Frank J. DellaCroce and The Center for Restorative Breast Surgery, LLC.

radiation frequently results in more complications and less satisfactory cosmetic results after immediate implant reconstruction with tissue expanders or implants.

Radiated skin sometimes doesn't recover sufficiently to swap the tissue expander for an implant, or the implant breaks through the damaged skin. In this case, the implant can remain in place and be covered with a flap of fat and muscle from the back, or it can be removed and replaced with a tissue flap. Small European studies show that padding the radiated mastectomy site with fat before placing the implant can reduce complications. Women who had *fat grafts* (chapter 10)—fat that was liposuctioned from their hips, thighs, or abdomen—and then had the fat injected into the radiated tissue had no complications after 15 to 17 months, and all of them were quite satisfied with their new breasts.[6]

Radiation can also affect flap reconstruction. The breast might feel harder, have a different skin color, or shrink as tissue contracts. A portion of the flap may die, and in rare cases, the entire flap may fail. Because flap procedures bring healthy tissue to the mastectomy site, they produce better results when they're performed after radiation. Several research projects have confirmed that delaying flap reconstruction for more than a year after radiation produces fewer complications and overall better shape and volume, particularly in the upper pole of the breast.[7]

Delayed-immediate reconstruction. If you're having mastectomy to treat invasive breast cancer, you may also need radiation, depending on the stage of your tumor and lymph node involvement. It's easier to plan the timing of your reconstruction if you know whether you need radiation before you go into surgery, but sometimes the need for adjuvant radiation isn't clear until post-mastectomy pathology results are available. For this reason, your surgeon may advise against immediate reconstruction if it's possible that you'll need radiation treatment. Delaying your reconstruction can be a hard pill to swallow, because it means you'll wake up from your mastectomy with a flat chest, and you'll miss the cosmetic benefits of immediate reconstruction. If you want to have reconstruction, you'll need to endure an additional surgery and recovery.

Delayed-immediate reconstruction is a unique approach to this issue that recognizes the immediate need for radiation therapy and provides the aesthetic advantages of immediate reconstruction (figure 3.6). After your breast tissue is removed, a tissue expander is placed under your chest muscle and fully inflated to preserve your breast shape and skin for later

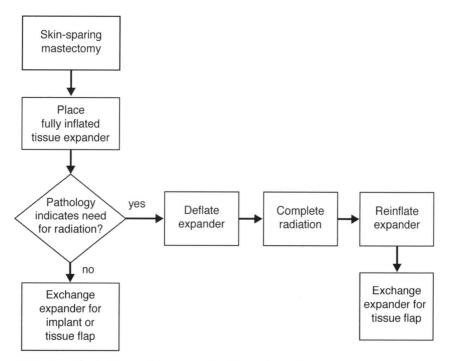

FIGURE 3.6. The decision-making process for delayed-immediate reconstruction.

reconstruction. If it turns out that you don't need radiation, you can proceed with reconstruction, swapping the expander for an implant or a tissue flap. If you do need radiation, the tissue expander can be deflated and left in place, then re-inflated a few months after your final radiation treatment. (Deflating expanders addresses the concern that expanders or implants may interfere with the precise delivery of radiation.) Several months later, you can proceed with tissue flap reconstruction—implants aren't generally advised, because of the high potential for complications following radiation therapy.

No standard guidelines dictate the timing of reconstruction when radiation is needed, and research hasn't produced enough large, long-term studies with definitive results one way or the other. Some plastic surgeons prefer to "try it and see what happens," while others proceed more conservatively. The truth is that radiation is unpredictable, and results differ from one woman to the next. Until advanced treatments can destroy tumors without damaging the surrounding tissue and skin, radiation will continue to influence reconstructive outcomes.

CHAPTER FOUR

How Mastectomy Affects Reconstruction

It was so important to me to come out of surgery looking essentially the same, and that is what keeping my own nipples did for me.   —ANDREA

If you're considering reconstruction, two questions are probably foremost in your mind: how will your new breasts look and how will they feel? Although reconstruction isn't perfect, and not all women have optimal outcomes, it can be a remarkable procedure. But even the best plastic surgeons can't replace what mastectomy takes away—your own natural breasts. Although mastectomy and reconstruction can be performed during one visit to the operating room, they're two distinct procedures by two different surgeons, and it's important to understand how one procedure influences the other.

Mastectomy Cause and Effect

Before your operation, your surgeon will draw the incision lines on your breast. If you have chosen to have immediate reconstruction with your mastectomy, he'll also mark around any previous biopsy scars where cancer was found; they'll be *re-excised* during surgery. This means cutting around the scar and removing it, just in case any cancerous cells remain. Each step of the mastectomy procedure affects your breast reconstruction.

Mastectomy action: Once you're asleep on the operating table, the surgeon makes incisions along the markings.

Effect: The placement of your incision(s) will depend on your breast size (how much tissue must be removed) and your plastic surgeon's preference to facilitate your reconstruction. Incisions leave permanent scars. Although your mastectomy scars may be hidden in the *inframammary fold* (the crease under your breast) or camouflaged by tattoos, incisions made on the front of the breast remain. Scars fade considerably within several months after surgery and become less visible after a year or two.

Mastectomy action: The surgeon removes the breast skin within the incisions, including the nipple and areola. There are exceptions to this practice, as you'll see later in this chapter.

Effect: New nipples can be created, but they will lack sensory nerve endings and won't respond to touch or cold as natural nipples do.

Effect: Amputating the nipple and areola and then closing the incision flattens the natural projection of the breast. The location or size of a tumor often requires removal of additional skin, which also reduces projection; projection is further reduced if more skin is removed from the front of the breast. Projection on the new breast tends to be better when the mastectomy incision runs vertically from the bottom of the areola to the inframammary fold, rather than horizontally across the nipple. Projection is also improved with immediate tissue flap reconstruction, which provides skin that replaces the missing nipple and areola. Using tissue expanders can also improve projection by expanding breast skin prior to placing the implant, especially if you keep your own nipples.

Mastectomy action: The surgeon separates the breast tissue from the underlying muscle and overlying skin, removing as much as possible—breast tissue runs from the collarbone to the underarm and across to the middle of the rib cage.

Effect: Because breast tissue blends with the thin layer of tissue beneath the skin and is intimately attached to the chest wall, it's not possible to remove all of it; some residual breast tissue is left behind, regardless of the type of mastectomy. That's why a small risk of recurrence remains after mastectomy.

Effect: Removing breast tissue eliminates milk ducts and lobules. Breast-feeding isn't possible after mastectomy, even if your breast and nipple are reconstructed, because you no longer have the mechanism to produce or deliver milk.

Effect: Removing breast tissue severs fine nerves that provide sensation to the skin, so much of the new breast will have little or no sensation. Nerves do regenerate slowly, typically growing about an inch per month, and more slowly after radiation or chemotherapy. Most women retain or recover some feeling in the upper, outer, and lower perimeters of their breasts and in between, but the front of the breast typically remains de-sensitized. Patches of pressure sensation may return after a year or more, but it won't be the same discrete sensitivity to touch, to cold, or to heat that you're used to. If you have immediate breast reconstruction that preserves most of your breast, more sensation may return, although this varies widely among mastectomy patients. As nerves regenerate, areas of your breasts may become hypersensitive—you might feel that you have too much sensation or have tingling, burning, or other strange sensations in your new breast. These unusual feelings gradually subside. Some women have *phantom sensations* similar to those experienced by people who lose an arm or a leg. For a while, your brain continues to receive sense impulses from nerves in the breast, even though the nerves have been severed or removed.

Younger women tend to regain more sensation, as do those who have flap reconstruction, which restores more sensation than implants because nerve endings in the chest often spontaneously connect with those in the flap. Improving sensation by attaching nerves in the flap to an intercostal nerve in the chest is an unpredictable process that requires meticulous skill and often isn't possible because the recipient nerve in the chest is damaged during mastectomy. It's been tried, but evidence supporting the success of this procedure has been anecdotal, and it is rarely attempted.

My reconstructed breasts look fabulous, but I can't feel a thing except along the outside. Most of my breasts feel as though they've been shot through with Novocain. When I'm sitting down, I can lean forward and not even feel the edge of the table pressing into my new boobs. They could be on fire, and I wouldn't know it! You get used to it. —Angel

I decided on a nipple-sparing mastectomy with immediate reconstruction because my breasts were important to my sexuality, and I was very concerned about losing erogenous sensation. I knew no procedure could guarantee my sensation would return, but I wanted the highest possibility. So when choosing my reconstruction, I searched until I found a surgeon who would also do nerve reconnection, despite the fact that it is controversial. It took a year and a half, but my right breast now has nearly normal sensation, and the nipple has some erogenous sensation. It's not as pleasurable as before, but it is thrilling to have some of the feeling back. My left breast has almost full sensation in the skin; although my nipple senses touch and temperature, it has no erogenous response. I know many women regain feeling without the added two-hour surgery I had to reconnect nerves, so it's hard to know if my sensation would have returned anyway. I feel lucky and just like the same old me, which was all I really wanted.   —Lisa

Skin-Sparing Procedures

If you have immediate reconstruction, a *skin-sparing mastectomy* will pre-serve most of your breast skin to hold an implant or a tissue flap. Your nipple and areola will be removed through a circular or elliptical ("cat's eye") incision, leaving a hole through which the entire mastectomy and reconstruction will be performed. An additional incision to the side or below the nipple may be needed to remove biopsy scars and breast tissue or to reach the lymph nodes (figure 4.1). During implant reconstruction, the opening is closed horizontally, laterally, or with *purse string sutures*—stitches that are threaded around the edges of the opening and pulled closed, similar to a gathering technique in sewing. The puckered scar will be covered by later nipple reconstruction and tattooing. Some surgeons prefer to fill the hole with a small skin graft taken from the stomach, thigh, or hip. If you have reconstruction with your own tissue, a portion of the flap skin will fill the opening.

Compared to delayed reconstruction, skin-sparing mastectomy with immediate reconstruction produces a new breast with minimal scarring. If

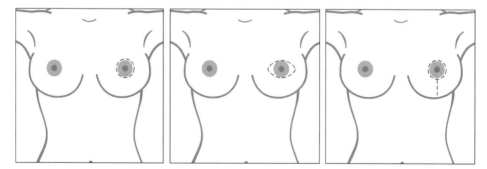

FIGURE 4.1. Skin-sparing mastectomy may be performed through a periareolar incision (*left*) or a cat's eye incision (*center*). An additional vertical or horizontal incision may also be required (*right*).

you begin mastectomy and immediate reconstruction without breast scars from previous biopsies or other operations, you have a good chance of emerging in much the same way. Skin-sparing mastectomies aren't recommended if you have inflammatory breast cancer or cancer in or near your breast skin.

Saving Your Nipple and Areola

Nipple-sparing mastectomy (*NSM*) represents the evolution of breast removal procedures: from Halsted's radical mastectomy that took the entire breast, chest muscles, and lymph nodes, to NSM that removes breast tissue but saves almost all of the entire visible breast, including skin, nipple, and areola. With your mastectomy scar well hidden, NSM produces the best cosmetic results. Although what lies beneath the skin is different, the exterior of your breast appears natural, intact, and virtually unchanged.

Removing breast tissue during mastectomy eliminates much of the blood supply that feeds the breast skin, including the nipple and areola. Compared to a skin-sparing mastectomy that removes the nipple and areola, a NSM requires extra skill and experience to carefully remove tissue at the base of the areola without damaging the delicate blood vessels that support the nipple. If this vital blood supply is compromised, some or the entire nipple may die. The odds of that happening are reduced when the mastectomy incision is made in the breast crease or along the outer contour, rather than around the nipple. Incisions may also be made from the areola down to the bottom of the breast or across to the outer breast (figure 4.2).

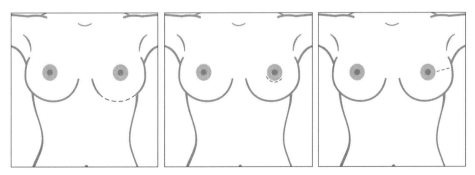

FIGURE 4.2. Nipple-sparing incisions are often made under the breast (*left*), beneath the areola (*center*), or to the side of the areola (*right*).

Some surgeons prefer a smaller incision at the base of the areola with or without an adjacent lateral incision.

Many surgeons use special imaging technology to assess the quality of blood flow to the nipple while you're still in the OR. (Blood flow that appears weak during surgery may subsequently improve.) Radiation therapy before or after NSM with immediate reconstruction increases the chance of necrosis, slow healing, and nipple loss but doesn't usually compromise nipple retention. Smoking also raises the risk of losing the nipple.[1] If the nipple dies, it must be removed, and a new one, if desired, can be recreated. Other factors, including whether you have circulatory problems, may also influence nipple survival.

Performing a minor *nipple delay* procedure in the weeks before the mastectomy can boost the chance that the nipple will survive the subsequent NSM. Usually performed in the office under local anesthesia, the breast surgeon makes an incision and separates the nipple and areola from the breast tissue below for about an inch or two around the entire areola. (The same incision will be reused during the mastectomy.) Disconnecting the blood supply from the underlying tissue encourages the nipple to use more of the blood vessels in the surrounding skin, which are stimulated to grow. A small sample of breast tissue is removed at the same time. If it is found to be clear of cancer cells, the NSM can proceed. If cancer cells are found in the tissue, a skin-sparing mastectomy will be done instead, and the nipple and areola will be removed.

During NSM, the nipple and areola remain attached to the breast. The underlying tissue at the base of the nipple is removed and examined; if cancer is found, the nipple is also removed. (NSM isn't the same as the *subcutaneous* mastectomies performed in the 1970s that intentionally left behind breast tissue—and sometimes cancer cells—to preserve adequate blood supply to the nipple.) Some surgeons core the interior of the nipple, replacing the tissue with a bit of rib cartilage or a synthetic surgical material; this leaves the nipple permanently erect. Not all surgeons do this, so it's worth asking about how your nipple-sparing procedure will be performed. Some experts believe that not coring the nipple slightly raises the risk for future cancer, but good evidence shows that the type of ductal-lobular structure where cancer typically develops isn't usually found in the nipple, and when cancer develops, it is usually found deeper in the breast.[2]

Although 20- to 30-year studies of recurrence rates after NSM aren't yet available, and medical experts haven't reached consensus on selection criteria, research shows that NSM is safe for carefully selected candidates who have small, non-aggressive tumors that aren't in the skin or close to the nipple, or women who have preventive mastectomy to reduce their inherited risk of breast cancer.[3]

If your reconstructed breast isn't the same size or shape as your natural breast, retained nipples may not be centered or where you want them, particularly after radiation. After unilateral mastectomy, the nipple on your reconstructed breast may not line up exactly with its counterpart on your opposite breast. Before reconstruction, ask your surgeon how he'll approach these issues and what you can realistically expect. If your breasts aren't overly large or don't sag extensively, your nipples are likely to end up where they should be after reconstruction: centered on your new breasts. If your breasts are *ptotic*, meaning they are oblong rather than round, and they head south so that the nipples point downward or hang below the inframammary fold, your surgeon might recommend skin-sparing rather than nipple-sparing mastectomy, because your nipples won't be well positioned after reconstruction. One way to get around the problem is to perform a breast lift (chapter 11) a few months after NSM and immediate tissue flap reconstruction to ensure proper nipple placement.[4] Alternatively, a breast reduction can be performed several weeks prior to mastectomy to better position your nipples after reconstruction.

Nipple banking is another nipple-sparing option that is more popular in Europe than in the United States. Nipples are removed during mastectomy and checked for cancerous cells. If they're clear, they are stored in the groin for several months until they can be transferred to the newly reconstructed and healed breast mounds. Banked nipples are flat and have little or no sensation.

What can you expect? If, like many women, you consider your nipples to be the focal point of your breasts, keeping them intact preserves a much-appreciated part of your natural breasts. But will they be the same? Cosmetic superiority aside, NSM is not without challenges and doesn't guarantee that your nipples will look, feel, or react as they did before. Unless the nipples are plumped with a piece of cartilage or a filler, they'll be flat. It's safe to say that most or all tactile sensation and erectile response to cold and touch will be lost, although it's difficult to predict if any will remain. A small subset of women report having almost full pre-mastectomy sensation after reconstruction. You have to wonder about that. Did their breast surgeon leave more tissue (and risk of recurrence) behind? It's hard to tell. Sensation is difficult to predict, because women retain or regain it to differing degrees, and not everyone perceives or defines it in the same way. Assessing the amount and quality of sensation is highly subjective, and is usually self-reported by patients. Even though sensation and response are considerably diminished after NSM, women often say it's a comfort to retain their own nipples. Others admit they wouldn't have chosen NSM if they knew in advance that their nipples wouldn't be the same.

Even though NSM isn't the standard of care, it's moved beyond the realm of experimental surgery. Not all physicians are on board with the concept, however, and many still prefer traditional remove-the-nipple procedures. Depending on your location, it may be difficult to find a breast surgeon or surgical oncologist who has experience with NSM.

Questions for your breast surgeon before nipple-sparing mastectomy:

- Am I a candidate for NSM?
- How many NSM procedures have you done?
- May I see photos of your reconstructions after nipple-sparing mastectomy?
- Where will my incisions be and how do they affect nipple reaction and sensation?
- How much sensation and reaction can I expect to retain?
- Do you remove the nipple or keep it attached during mastectomy?
- Will you check my nipple for cancer or abnormal cells during surgery?
- If I keep my nipples, will they be flat?
- Will my nipples be centered on my reconstructed breasts?
- What complications might occur and how will you address them?

I decided not to keep my nipples, because I inherited a very nasty family mutation, and my father developed breast cancer very near his nipple. I just told the doctor to "take everything." At 51 years old, I still had a pretty good intimate life with my husband, and I was not going to sacrifice my life for those nipples.   —*Debra*

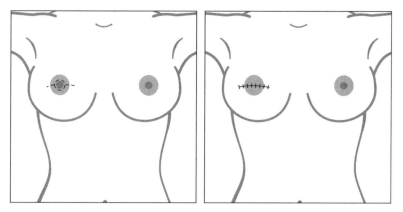

FIGURE 4.3. An areola-sparing mastectomy removes the nipple and breast tissue through an incision made across the areola.

Right after my nipple-sparing surgery my breasts were bruised and dented, with the nipples pointing in opposite directions. Week by week the bruising disappeared and the nipples evened out. After a few months, I was very pleased with my results, and within six months I was thrilled. It took about a year for my breasts to settle permanently. Now the scars under my breasts have faded to practically nothing. I went from an A-cup to a small C-cup, my projection looks natural, and I can go braless without a problem. It was so important to me to come out of surgery looking essentially the same, and that is what keeping my own nipples did for me. My new breasts look like my own and are fantastic! In fact, I'm happier with my breasts now than I was before surgery. I do not have any sensation on or around my nipples; however, I went into surgery well aware of this probability, and I accept it as part of the trade-off to vastly reduce my breast cancer risk. I would make the same decision, with the same surgeons, in a heartbeat. —Andrea

Areola-sparing mastectomy. Keeping your nipples isn't advised if you have a high risk for recurrence, but you may be able to keep your areolae if that appeals to you. Unlike nipples, areolae contain only skin cells. In an *areola-sparing mastectomy*, your breast tissue and nipple are removed with a horizontal incision across the areola (figure 4.3). A new nipple can be made later from the areola skin. Short-term studies show this procedure has few complications and doesn't significantly increase the odds of recurrence.

CHAPTER FIVE

Considering Prophylactic Mastectomy

*I do think prophylactic bilateral mastectomy is pretty
extreme, but so is cancer.* —JILL

Ironically, in some ways we've come full circle with regard to mastectomy. In an era of early detection and breast conservation, more *previvors*—women who inherit a high risk for breast cancer but haven't been diagnosed with the disease—are choosing to remove their healthy breasts.

Although scientists haven't found all the reasons that breast cancer runs in some families, the discovery of the *BReast CAncer1* (*BRCA1*) and the *BReast CAncer2* (*BRCA2*) genes introduced unprecedented insight into the biology of hereditary breast cancer. Although we often hear about people who decide to be tested to see whether they have the "breast cancer gene," this term is a misnomer. We all have two copies of BRCA1 and BRCA2 genes that, when healthy, produce proteins that repair cell damage and suppress tumor growth. Breast cancers are caused by *genetic mutations* inherited or acquired from lifestyle behaviors or environmental triggers as we age. When these abnormalities develop in BRCA genes, their protective function is lost, and the risk for developing breast and ovarian cancers increases significantly. Only 5 to 10 percent of breast cancers are thought to be hereditary; about half of these are caused by inherited mutations in BRCA1 or BRCA2 passed from one generation to the next. Either parent can pass on a BRCA mutation to their children—your children have a 50 percent chance of inheriting your mutation. Abnormalities in additional genes, including PALB2, CHEK2, ATM, BRIP1, and others, also increase hereditary cancer risk. (Other, as yet unidentified genes may also affect risk.) Having a family history of cancer, even when family members test negative for known mutations, can also elevate cancer risk.

Should You Have Genetic Testing?

Media reports often highlight how a small sample of an individual's blood can be used to trace ancestry, identify DNA in crime scene evidence, and determine genetic predisposition to disease. You might wonder whether you, too, should be tested for a genetic predisposition. *Genetic testing* is the only way to tell whether you've inherited a mutation that makes you prone to breast cancer. But testing isn't right for everyone, and not all families with breast cancer test positive for a mutation in a cancer-causing gene. Most, in fact, have negative test results.

If you're concerned that the cancer in your family is inherited, and you're considering genetic testing to see whether you carry a mutation, it's always a good idea to first consult with a health professional who is trained in cancer genetics. Consulting with a specially trained *genetic counselor* is an important first step. Using your personal and family medical history, she'll determine whether your family has a pattern of hereditary cancer, explain the benefits and limitations of genetic testing, and determine whether it's appropriate for you or other family members. If you test positive for a mutation, she'll explain how different risk management actions can reduce your chance of diagnosis. If your test is negative, she'll help you to understand the implications of that result. If your oncologist, surgeon, or other physician offers genetic testing but isn't trained to provide genetic counseling, ask for a referral to a qualified genetic counselor or genetics expert. Or check online to find a counselor by visiting the National Society of Genetic Counselors' website (www.nsgc.org) or using the National Cancer Institute's online directory (www.cancer.gov/cancertopics/genetics /directory). If no genetics experts are nearby or convenient, Informed Medical Decisions (www.informeddna.com) provides genetic counseling by telephone.

How Real Is Your Risk?

Saying that breast cancer risk is a complex subject is a gross understatement. Although researchers continue to make great strides in understanding the disease, much about it remains an enigma. The science of risk assessment is far from perfect, and too many unknowns prevent genetics experts from predicting who will or won't get breast cancer or accurately pinpointing an individual's exact level of risk.

For the average woman in the United States, breast cancer risk is based on the rate of diagnosis among the entire population; hence, the familiar 1-in-8 statistic. Calculating risk for someone who has a BRCA mutation is not as simple. For this, experts use estimates based on studies of breast cancer rates among high-risk families. Because these studies have found varying levels of risk, a high-risk individual's probability of developing breast cancer is typically expressed as a range of estimated risk. Because every person's situation is unique, your own risk assessment is influenced by the type of mutation you have, the risk factors that you can control (smoking, weight, birth control, breast-feeding, and others), and those you cannot (race, gender, age, family history, and others).

Regardless of the imprecise nature of risk assessment, experts agree on one premise: having a BRCA mutation or a strong family history of the disease doesn't guarantee that you'll one day be diagnosed with cancer, but it significantly raises your risk. The chance that you'll develop breast cancer at some point during your life is exceptionally high: 55 to 65 percent by age 70 if you have a BRCA1 mutation, and about 45 percent by age 70 if you have a mutation in BRCA2 (the average woman's 1-in-8 risk translates to about 12 percent).[1] New generations of women appear to be developing BRCA-related cancers at a younger age, perhaps due to the impacts of lifestyle and behavioral factors.[2] If you're a breast cancer survivor with a BRCA mutation, your risk of recurrence and another primary tumor is also greater. If you have a strong family history of cancer and test negative for a BRCA mutation, your risk is thought to be greater than that for a woman in the general population but less than the risk for someone who has a BRCA gene mutation. Mutations in several genes are associated with higher risk for certain cancers. If you are a woman with a BRCA gene mutation, you have a higher-than-average risk for:

- developing breast cancer
- diagnosis at a younger age
- breast cancer in both breasts
- other cancers, including ovarian cancer, pancreatic cancer, and melanoma

Men with mutations in BRCA1 or BRCA2 have increased risk for cancers of the breast, prostate, and pancreas. Having a BRCA2 mutation also raises a man's risk for melanoma.

Understanding high cancer risk can be perplexing, and confronting it is frightening; yet, both actions are opportunities to do something about it. Someday scientists may discover ways to repair defective genes. Until that time, if you're predisposed to developing breast cancer, you have options to manage your high risk:

- Increased surveillance with more frequent breast exams, mammograms, and other screenings. These actions don't lower the risk of developing cancer but they may detect a future breast cancer at an early, more treatable stage.
- Risk-reducing medication (with increased surveillance).
- Preventive surgery.

Preventive Surgeries That Reduce Your Risk

If you're a previvor, *prophylactic bilateral mastectomy* (PBM) is the most effective way to reduce your breast cancer risk, lowering the odds of a diagnosis by 90 percent or more.[3] (A small risk remains because it's impossible to remove every bit of breast tissue.) If your estimated risk for breast cancer is 65 percent, PBM will reduce that to about 6 to 7 percent, lower than the risk for women who don't have a BRCA mutation or a strong family history of breast cancer. (Other lifestyle and behavioral factors can also increase or further decrease your level of risk.)

Some experts argue that many women who remove their breasts do so needlessly, because not all of them would ever develop breast cancer. Clinically, that may be an understandable position. You might not have the same point of view, though, if you're extraordinarily prone to developing breast cancer or you've seen loved ones struggle with a cancer diagnosis and treatment, and you would do just about anything to avoid the same fate. Even with its impressive risk-reducing benefit, PBM is a deeply personal choice. Despite increasing media stories about the surgery, including accounts by high-profile celebrities, it isn't right for everyone, and it shouldn't be considered lightly, because once it's done, it can't be undone.

TABLE 5.1. Reducing breast cancer risk with preventive surgery

Procedure(s)	Estimated risk reduction (%)
Bilateral preventive mastectomy	90*
Bilateral salpingo-oophorectomy (before natural menopause)	53
Both surgeries	95

*For women with intact ovaries.

However, if you're prepared to do whatever you can to reduce your high chance of being diagnosed with breast cancer and dealing with mastectomy, chemotherapy, or radiation, it's your most effective alternative.

PBM may be an easy decision for some women. Others would never consider removing their healthy breasts. Whatever your circumstances, the decision can be torturous. Should you? Shouldn't you? No one can answer that question for you. If you decide PBM is the best way to have peace of mind as you live your life, you'll be a candidate for skin-sparing or nipple-sparing mastectomies with immediate reconstruction. From a cosmetic standpoint, reconstruction after PBM produces some of the very best results, particularly if your healthy breasts are unscarred from biopsies or previous surgeries. If you're unsatisfied with the shape, size, or position of your natural breasts, reconstruction can correct those issues, even though your new breasts won't have the same sensation.

If you have a BRCA mutation, experts also recommend preventive *bilateral salpingo-oophorectomy (BSO)*—removal of both ovaries—between ages 35 and 40 or when you complete childbearing. BSO before natural menopause reduces ovarian cancer risk by 80 percent and lowers breast cancer risk by half (table 5.1).[4] Both PBM and BSO lower overall breast cancer risk by 95 percent and offer an additional benefit: if you develop breast cancer after BSO, your odds of a second diagnosis are cut in half.[5] The decision to have BSO should be made only after careful consideration, because it can cause serious side effects. If you're still having menstrual periods, it will push your body into menopause, and you may prematurely experience hot flashes, insomnia, vaginal dryness, and other change-of-life symptoms. Your gynecologist or oncologist can discuss these issues with you and let you know what to expect.

My mother has breast cancer again; one of her sisters is in stage 4, another is in remission. My grandmother and the rest of my mother's sisters died of cancer. Even with this history, having my breasts removed was the hardest decision I've ever had to make. Though I had many breakdowns, I knew after all the crying that the decision I made was the right one. My breasts were precious to me but not as precious as my children. I wanted to make sure I'll be here to see them go off to life. Believe me when I say it's a relief. —Nora

I do think prophylactic bilateral mastectomy is pretty extreme, but so is cancer. It's all a matter of how much risk you are willing to live with day to day, compared to your willingness to undergo major surgery to reduce that risk to as close to zero as possible. You do as much research as you can by reading and talking to people who have the appropriate knowledge and experience, then you do what's right for you. I didn't want PBM. However, in examining my own personal and family history, my temperament, and life goals, I couldn't not have it. —Jill

Ultimately, whether or not you proceed with prophylactic mastectomy is your decision, but everyone you know will have an opinion about what you should or shouldn't do. Friends and family might consider breast removal to be extreme. Unless they've had to make the decision themselves, people may not comprehend why you would deliberately remove your perfectly healthy breasts. They might not understand that while you would certainly prefer to keep your breasts, you view them as life-threatening enemies.

Take the time you need to consider what each risk-reducing option involves, how it affects your current and future level of risk, and potential side effects. Speak with your health care team, including a genetics specialist, to gain a clear sense of your own risk. Carefully consider your tolerance for risk, your lifestyle, and other factors before deciding which alternative is the best decision for you. Facing Our Risk of Cancer Empowered (FORCE), the foremost nonprofit education and support group for people with hereditary cancer, provides information online (www.facingourrisk.org), by phone, and through outreach coordinators in most states. The organization's message boards offer a supportive, safe, and empowering place to learn, share, and just vent about genetic high risk, prophylactic surgery, mastectomy, and reconstruction. *Confronting Hereditary Breast and Ovarian Cancer*, the organization's decision-making resource for previvors and survivors of hereditary cancer, is a comprehensive roadmap for living in a high-risk body.

Paying for Preventive High-Risk Services

If you test positive for an inherited mutation that raises your risk of breast cancer, most health insurers will cover the costs for recommended increased surveillance, risk-reducing medication, and preventive mastectomy with or without reconstruction. Out-of-pocket expenses depend on the specific service performed and the details of your policy. If your request for coverage is denied, ask your primary care physician, oncologist, or medical geneticist to write a supportive letter explaining how your high-risk status meets nationally recognized guidelines for these services. The FORCE website has several sample appeal letters.

PART TWO ○ RECONSTRUCTIVE PROCEDURES

CHAPTER SIX

Breast Implants

I don't mind if the implant must be exchanged in the future.
I consider it required maintenance, like getting my car
serviced. —BELLE

In the early days of modern breast reconstruction, implants were the only method of replacing breast tissue. It's still the simplest method of reconstruction and compared with tissue flap procedures, it is shorter, not as invasive, leaves fewer scars, and doesn't require the special surgical skills required with tissue flaps. Recovery is faster, but generally, the traditional overall reconstruction process takes longer to complete.

Implant reconstruction is a good option if you:

- don't have an active infection anywhere in your body
- aren't pregnant or nursing
- don't want to scar additional areas of your body
- don't have enough fat for a tissue flap reconstruction
- can't endure a lengthier flap reconstruction operation
- are willing to surgically alter your healthy breast to achieve symmetry (an option if you have unilateral reconstruction)

Implants Inside and Out

Implant reconstruction is the most common method of rebuilding breasts, accounting for about 80 percent of procedures. It involves several decisions that are best made during consultation with your plastic surgeon, who will describe where your incisions will be made and explain the different types of implants available to you.

Saline or silicone? Breast implants are filled with either *saline* (sterile salt water) or *silicone* gel. Both have outer shells of medical-grade silicone rubber. A breast reconstructed with a saline implant lacks the softness, resilience, and bounce of silicone gel, which behaves and feels more like natural breast tissue. In the 1970s and 1980s, silicone implants were filled with a thinner type of silicone. The interior of fourth-generation silicone implants is similar to honey. Fifth-generation models contain *highly cohesive gel* that is semi-solid like Jell-O; these "gummy bear" implants are firm yet soft and are said to be "form stable"—they maintain the teardrop shape. Although not without potential issues, compared to their earlier counterparts, highly cohesive gel implants are thought to have fewer complications, are less likely to rupture, and last longer. These improvements, combined with shorter surgery and recovery than tissue flap reconstruction, make silicone implants quite popular: about 75 percent of all reconstruction with breast implants use silicone devices.[1] After reconstruction, women with silicone implants report significantly higher satisfaction than women with saline implants, and rates of complications and satisfaction with silicone implants are similar, regardless of the manufacturer.[2]

During your consultation appointment, ask to see and hold both types of implants so you can compare how they feel. (Some surgeons only use one kind or the other.) Speak with other women who have had implant reconstruction (your plastic surgeon can put you in touch), so you'll have the benefit of their experience. Consider the advantages and disadvantages of silicone and saline before you make your final decision about how your reconstruction will be done (table 6.1).

Shape and texture. Breast implants are either round or contoured (figure 6.1). (Contoured implants are also often referred to as "teardrop" or "anatomical.") Round implants create fullness across the breast. When you stand or sit, saline collects in the lower portion of the implant, providing a natural slope to the breast. When you lie flat, it moves toward the outside of the breast, as natural tissue does. Contoured implants are longer and narrower, with more fullness at the bottom. You might think they would provide a more natural shape, but they aren't always the best solution. Your chest dimensions influence the shape of your new breast as much as, if not more than, the type of implant used, and contoured im-

TABLE 6.1. Comparing saline and silicone implants

Characteristic	Saline implant	Silicone implant
Components	Silicone shell filled with salt water	Silicone shell filled with silicone gel
Texture	Firm, like a water balloon	Soft, more like breast tissue
Interior	Filled by surgeon during operation	Pre-filled by manufacturer
Incision required	Shorter (implant is deflated when inserted)	Longer (implant is full when inserted)
Rupture	Obvious	May be undetected
Follow-up recommended	None	Periodic MRI screening

plants, which must fit more exactly to the chest, are not a good fit for all women. They have a rough, textured exterior that adheres to the surrounding scar tissue, so they're less likely to shift or rotate in the pocket and distort breast shape. This is less of an issue with round implants, which retain their shape even when they move in the pocket.

Textured breast implants were developed to discourage *capsular contracture,* hard scar tissue that squeezes the implant and can distort its shape. This doesn't always work, however, and *rippling*—indentations that look like small waves under the skin—occurs more frequently in textured implants. Texturing also creates a thicker implant wall, so it's more likely that you'll be able to see or feel the edges of your implant. Your plastic surgeon will help you decide which shape and type of implant best fits your needs.

Size and projection. Communicating how big or small you'd like your new breasts to be isn't as easy as saying "make me a 36B," because implant volume doesn't readily translate to bra size. Implant capacity is measured in cubic centimeters (cc): 30 cc equals one ounce. Your physical characteristics

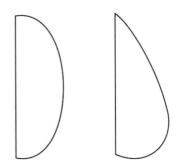

FIGURE 6.1. Implants are either round (*left*) or contoured (*right*).

make all the difference in how a particular implant looks in proportion to the rest of your body: a 480 cc implant will look much larger on a 5′ 4″ woman who weighs 120 pounds than on a woman who is 5′ 9″ and weighs 160 pounds.

If you have unilateral reconstruction, your surgeon will choose an implant that closely matches the size of your opposite breast. (If you prefer smaller or larger breasts, your healthy breast can be modified with one of the procedures described in chapter 11.) With bilateral reconstruction, you have a clean slate for new breasts that are smaller, bigger, or similar to your natural breast. Choosing the right size is important. Implants that are too small won't give you the volume you want, and if they're too large, they might upset your body's aesthetic proportions. Many women leave the choice of implants to their surgeons. However, the size of your reconstructed breast shouldn't be a surprise. By actively participating in the decision, you're more likely to be satisfied with the size of your reconstructed breasts. Dissatisfaction with size is a common reason for replacing implants, so it's a good idea to be sure you and your surgeon are on the same page about what you want.

 Your surgeon will select implants that fit the diameter of your chest wall and, among those, will choose one that provides the volume and projection you want. If you're large-framed, low- or moderate-profile implants, which are wider at the base, will provide a better fit than high-profile implants that have more projection but are designed to fit women with a narrow chest (figure 6.2).

ADVANTAGES OF IMPLANT RECONSTRUCTION
- *Surgery and recovery are shorter and less complex than tissue flap reconstruction.*
- *It reuses the mastectomy incision for reconstruction without additional scarring.*
- *The procedure can be completed in a single step when combined with nipple-sparing mastectomy (if no revisions are required).*

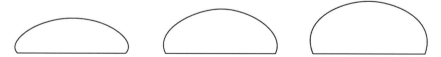

FIGURE 6.2. Implants are available in different widths, volumes, and profiles.

- *It is a viable alternative for women who don't want or can't have flap reconstruction.*
- *Future weight changes won't affect the size of your new breasts.*
- *It's easy to find qualified surgeons.*

DISADVANTAGES OF IMPLANT RECONSTRUCTION

- *The overall reconstruction process can be much longer than a tissue flap procedure.*
- *Most procedures involve multiple steps and multiple office visits.*
- *The new breast doesn't feel, look, or move like living tissue.*
- *Implants are subject to rupture, deflation, capsular contracture, and other inherent problems that may require reoperation and replacement.*
- *Results are often poor in radiated tissue.*
- *Surgical modification of the healthy breast is usually needed to achieve symmetry after unilateral reconstruction.*
- *Implants don't last a lifetime.*

Are They Safe?

Breast implants have been around in one form or another since the early 1960s. By the time the U.S. Food and Drug Administration (FDA) began regulating implants in 1976, thousands of women already had them. Lawsuits filed in the 1990s claimed that silicone implants caused arthritis, immune system disorders, and a host of other health problems. Implant companies and plastic surgeons were caught between a rock and a hard place: though implants had been used for 30 years, their long-term safety had never been established. Although no scientific evidence linked silicone breast implants to any significant health problems, in 1992 the FDA banned use of the devices for cosmetic purposes, reclassified them as experimental, and approved their use only for breast reconstruction and clinical studies until manufacturers could prove the devices were safe. The Institute of Medicine studied the issue comprehensively, concluding in 1999 that "a review of toxicology studies of silicones and other substances known to be in breast implants does not provide a basis for health concerns."[3] Subsequent studies in the United States, Canada, and Europe concurred. With no evidence of a cause-and-effect relationship between silicone breast implants and health concerns, the FDA reversed the ban in 2006. Breast implants are regulated in the United States, and every woman with a silicone implant becomes part of a national database used to track and evaluate problems.

Silicone breast implants are the most-studied medical devices in the history of medicine, and potential problems aside, they're considered to be safe. Medical-grade silicone is the most common material used in artificial joints, pacemakers, and other devices that are placed in the body. A small percentage of women with silicone implants develop characteristics of lupus, psoriasis, chronic fatigue syndrome, rheumatoid arthritis, and other autoimmune conditions. Scientists point out that these symptoms occur no more frequently in women who have silicone implants than in women who don't. Some experts still believe that silicone may be problematic for women who already have weakened immune systems. Women with breast implants may have a very low but increased risk of developing *anaplastic large cell lymphoma* (*ALCL*), a rare type of non-Hodgkin lymphoma that can develop adjacent to or in the scar tissue surrounding the implant.[4] The FDA recommends seeing a physician if the area around an implant looks or feels unusual.

Tissue Expander-to-Implant Reconstruction

Implant reconstruction is either a one-step or two-step procedure. Most women have a two-step process with temporary implants called *tissue expanders*. Placed in the body, expanders slowly stretch tissues and create new skin, similar to the way a woman's belly expands during pregnancy. It's a safe and effective way to replace large areas of severely burned skin, repair other physical deformities, and prepare the post-mastectomy chest to receive implants. For breast reconstruction, the first step places expanders beneath the pectoralis major muscle. The expanders are gradually inflated until the skin and muscle have stretched enough to accommodate a full-sized breast implant (the second step).

You might wonder why expansion is necessary, considering that women who have breast augmentation to enlarge their healthy breasts don't need it. They have breast tissue and skin that can accommodate an implant; after mastectomy, that breast tissue is gone, and the remaining breast skin is thinner. Tissue expansion is beneficial for women with very thin or problematic skin, including smokers and those who have had radiation to the breast. (It's also necessary for delayed implant reconstruction, because most of the breast skin has been removed.) A newer, more streamlined technique places the implant in a single procedure, but most surgeons prefer the reliability and effectiveness of the traditional two-stage method: 90 percent of breast reconstruction with implants involve tissue expansion.[5]

Creating a pocket. Working through the mastectomy incision, the surgeon detaches the lower edge of the muscle from the chest wall, then lifts the muscle and shapes a pocket behind it. A deflated expander is placed in the pocket; the muscle edge is then pulled down over the upper portion of the expander, and the incision is closed. Initially, the expander is partially filled with 60 to 100 cc or more of saline. This pushes the muscle forward, creating a small bulge. The process takes about an hour for each breast. When you wake up, you'll have starter breast mounds, so your chest won't be completely flat. Over several weeks the expander stretches the muscle until the pocket is large enough to hold the implant (figure 6.3).

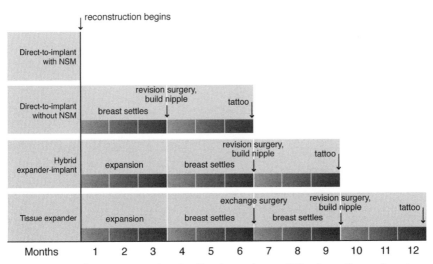

FIGURE 6.3. Implant reconstruction timeline. Intervals may differ, depending on breast cancer treatment, the preference of patient and surgeon, and complications that may delay completion.

Expansion and implant exchange. In about three or four weeks, when your chest has healed sufficiently, your surgeon will gradually add saline to slowly inflate your expanders. This constant pressure thins the chest muscle and enlarges the pocket. At the same time, it pushes the muscle against the front of the breast, stretching the skin. When the sub-muscular pocket is large enough, you'll have a short exchange surgery to replace the expanders with softer and better-shaped saline or silicone implants. (Expansion is described in more detail in chapter 7.)

After several weeks, when your implants have settled into place, your new nipple can be created in a short operation (chapter 12). Cosmetic revisions, if required, can also be performed at this stage. The final, separate step in the reconstructive process adds color to the nipple and simulates the areola.

Direct-to-Implant Reconstruction

Direct-to-implant reconstruction (also called *non-expansive, one-step,* and *single-stage* reconstruction) places a full-sized implant into the pocket immediately after mastectomy, eliminating the need for expansion. Unless complications occur or revisions are necessary, this skip-a-step procedure completes the entire "invisible" reconstruction during a single visit to the operating room. You're a candidate for this procedure if you have a nipple-sparing mastectomy that retains enough breast skin to cover the implant. Unlike expansion, direct-to-implant reconstruction doesn't require exchange surgery or nipple reconstruction. An *acellular dermal matrix (ADM),* a sterile tissue substitute made from human cadaver, swine, or bovine skin that has been stripped of its cells but retains collagen and other proteins, facilitates direct-to-implant reconstruction. Adding a patch of the material along the edge of the muscle covers the lower portion of the implant (figure 6.4), creating an internal bra that holds the implant in position, thereby completing in a single procedure what expansion achieves over several weeks. (While placing implants beneath the muscle is the preferred method for breast reconstruction, some surgeons place the implant over the muscle, cushioning it from the skin with a layer of ADM.) The ADM also partially replaces tissue lost during mastectomy, smoothing breast contour and cushioning the skin from direct contact

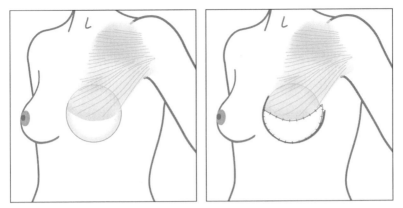

FIGURE 6.4. In traditional implant reconstruction, the pectoralis muscle covers only the upper part of the implant (*left*). Adding a patch of acellular dermal matrix along the lower edge of the muscle (*right*) provides complete coverage of the implant.

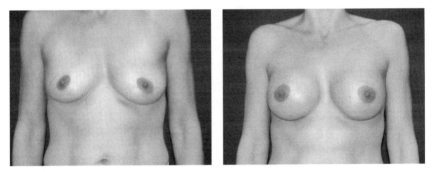

FIGURE 6.5. Before (*left*) and after (*right*) bilateral nipple-sparing mastectomy with immediate direct-to-implant reconstruction. Images provided by C. Andrew Salzberg, M.D.

with the implant. Originally developed as *skin grafts* for burn victims, acellular material is organic, providing a biological framework that supports the growth of new blood vessels. AlloDerm, Tutoplast, DermaMatrix, Strattice, Seri-Silk (made of silk), and other ADMs are regulated by the FDA.

If direct-to-implant reconstruction (figure 6.5) appeals to you, consider the following:

- Most surgeons still prefer the tried-and-true expansion process, so it may be difficult to find someone who offers this streamlined method of implant reconstruction.
- Choose a plastic surgeon who is well experienced with the procedure.

- Verify that a plastic surgeon performs direct-to-implant reconstruction, because many plastic surgeons use ADM with traditional expansion reconstruction to provide additional soft coverage over the implant.
- Women who have ADMs with tissue expanders may be more prone to infections at the surgical site than women who have tissue expanders without ADMs.[6]
- Reconstruction that begins as direct-to-implant may require additional procedures to correct problems or improve cosmetic results.
- Eligibility for direct-to-implant reconstruction requires healthy breast skin. Ask your surgeon whether you're a candidate.

Choosing preventive mastectomy to reduce my inherited risk for breast cancer was a difficult decision. I did not think I would be able to look in the mirror if I had no reconstruction, but I knew I did not want to have fat removed from other parts of my body and endure more scars and healing time. I wanted my reconstruction to be over and done; I did not want to have to go back for fills and more surgery. Then I discovered nipple-sparing mastectomy with direct-to-implant reconstruction. The surgery was minimal and recovery was short. My procedure was a success, and three or four weeks later, I felt very good. I was an A-cup before my mastectomy; now I am a B-cup. I look so much better than before, and I have sensation toward the outer parts of my breasts. My nipples react to cold, yet I have no feeling on or around them. I love the results.   *—Leslie*

Two other immediate procedures bypass the traditional expansion process. Small-breasted women who have enough skin after mastectomy may be able to accommodate a fixed-volume implant right away, without expansion or exchange procedures. Women who have reconstruction that covers a breast implant with a tissue flap can also skip tissue expansion.

Recovery

After implant reconstruction, your chest will be numb and may feel heavy or ache for several days. If lymph nodes were removed during your sur-

TABLE 6.2. Intervals for implant reconstruction and recovery

Procedure	Surgery and hospital stay	Most routine activities resumed
Mastectomy and expanders	About 1–2 hours per breast; usually 1 day in hospital*	4–6 weeks
Exchange surgery	Up to 1 hour per breast; outpatient	1 week
Mastectomy and direct-to-implant	About 2 hours per breast; 1 day in hospital*	2–3 weeks

Note: Reflects bilateral reconstruction without complications. Surgical expertise and individual healing affect recovery times.
*Delayed reconstruction can be performed as an outpatient procedure.

gery, your underarm may also be numb or sore. Any discomfort will be controlled by pain medication. You'll be encouraged to get up and begin walking the day after your surgery. You should take progressively longer walks each day, and perform the exercises recommended by your surgeon to gradually improve your range of motion. You'll be tired and sore for a couple of weeks, but your strength will slowly return. Each day, you'll spend more time awake and less time napping. You may need to restrict upper body motion for a week or longer, and for several weeks you should avoid strenuous activities and movements that pull excessively on the muscle (table 6.2).

Before reconstruction, you may wonder whether you'll always be conscious of your implants. Will they ever feel a part of you, as your natural breasts did? They may feel heavy at first, and you'll feel them shift in the pocket when you stretch or lift, and move when your chest muscles flex or contract. This shouldn't be painful, although it can feel odd until you become accustomed to it. After several months, your implants will become softer, feel better, and drop into a more natural position on your chest. You'll get used to them in time.

Bras are optional after implant reconstruction. Even though you won't need one, you might enjoy wearing lingerie after reconstruction. If you decide to shop for new bras, you may need a different size than you wore before your mastectomy, because your new breasts may not have the same shape, size, or projection. You may be limited to wearing seamless stretch or lightly padded bras if your breast doesn't project enough to fill a regular bra cup, particularly if your nipples were removed. After unilateral reconstruction, it may be difficult to find a bra that fits both breasts correctly, unless your healthy breast is modified to achieve symmetry.

Potential Problems

Though many women who have implants are quite satisfied, complications, including many that require revision surgery, are not uncommon. You can find information online, including the type and frequency of complications, for each manufacturer's device. Search for "Labeling for Approved Breast Implants" at www.fda.gov/breastimplants or check the implant manufacturer's website. Or ask your plastic surgeon for a copy of the implant packaging; it's the same information.

Ruptures and leaks. A *rupture* is a tear in the outer shell of an implant that can result from injury to the breast, normal aging of the implant, or other reasons. Newer implants are more durable, potentially decreasing the frequency of ruptures and leaks; yet, they can still occur. The Ideal implant (www.idealimplant.com) features a unique design of nested, saline-filled chambers. Developed with input from plastic surgeons, it's designed to decrease ruptures and wrinkles, while providing a more natural feel, much like a silicone implant.

If a saline implant leaks, your reconstructed breast will deflate in a very obvious way (figure 6.6). The body safely absorbs the harmless saline, but the implant must be removed. When a silicone implant ruptures, you might feel a hard knot; have breast pain, swelling, or numbness; or notice a change in your breast size or shape. Because the cohesive gel usually remains in the pocket or scar capsule around it, you may be unaware of the rupture. If an MRI, ultrasound, or *computed tomography* (*CT*) scan shows that the implant has indeed ruptured, it must be removed and can then be replaced. Because there are often no visual changes to indicate the *silent rupture* of a silicone implant, the FDA recommends an MRI three years after your initial implant surgery and every two years thereafter (your health insurance may not pay for these screenings). Visit YouTube (www.youtube.com) and search for "breast implant rupture" if you'd like to see how punctures or ruptures affect saline and silicone implants.

Capsular contracture. After reconstruction, a capsule of scar tissue forms around the implant. This isn't unusual and it isn't a health hazard. It's the body's natural reaction to foreign matter and also occurs in patients who have pacemakers, artificial hips,

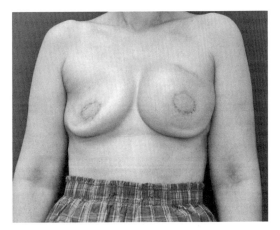

FIGURE 6.6. Although a silicone rupture may go unnoticed, a saline implant rupture, as shown here, is obvious. Image provided by Gail S. Lebovic, MA, MD, FACS.

or other types of implants. Capsular contracture—the most common reason for reoperation after implant reconstruction—occurs when scar tissue thickens, tightens, and squeezes the implant. Experts believe this condition probably develops when bacterial infection occurs in the scar capsule or when fluid or blood stimulates the growth of scar tissue around the implant. Mild capsular contracture (grades I and II) may cause the breast to feel more firm without affecting its appearance. More severe cases (grades III and IV) can be painful and distort the breast, pushing it high on the chest (figure 6.7). The condition develops more commonly in smokers and in women who have had radiation, though it's a mystery why some

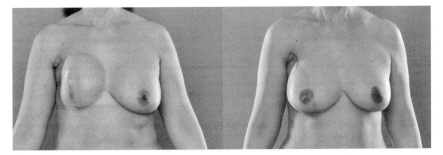

FIGURE 6.7. Capsular contracture may distort breast shape (*left*). This delayed reconstruction was salvaged by removing the scar tissue and replacing the implant with a tissue flap (*right*). Images provided by Dr. Frank J. DellaCroce and The Center for Restorative Breast Surgery, LLC.

women experience capsular contracture repeatedly, or develop it in one breast and not the other, and other women never experience it. It can develop within a few months of reconstruction or years later.

The best defense for capsular contracture is a good offense. Using textured implants, placing the implant beneath the muscle, or using an ADM may help to prevent capsular contracture, but they don't guarantee that it won't occur. Your surgeon can also show you how to massage your implants to discourage formation of additional scar tissue. Observing a "no touch" technique in the operating room to reduce infection around the implant can also help. Before placing the implant into the pocket, the surgeon changes his surgical gown and bathes his gloves, surgical instruments, and the implant in antibiotic liquid. The sub-muscular pocket is also flushed with antibiotic liquid. The aim is to reduce the level of bacteria on the surface of the implant before it goes into the chest.

If capsular contracture does cause problems, your surgeon may recommend an anti-inflammatory medication, vitamin E, ultrasound massage, or physical therapy. For more severe cases, the remedy involves *capsulectomy*, surgical removal of the scar capsule. (*Capsulotomy*, cutting into the capsule to release the scar formation, is associated with a high risk of recurring capsular contracture and is not generally considered to be an effective solution.) If the implant is removed and replaced, using an ADM with a replacement implant may help to deter another capsular contracture, perhaps by reducing inflammation around the implant, but there's no guarantee it won't happen again.[7] Muscle relaxants may also help. A different approach to the problem was discovered when asthma patients noticed that their scars improved. As a result, two asthma medications, Accolate and Singulair, are sometimes prescribed off-label to reduce capsular contracture. These medications can cause moderate to serious side effects, however, and no long-term studies of their effectiveness for this purpose have been conducted.

Rippling or wrinkling. You may be able to feel or see ripples or wrinkles in your implant, especially if your breast skin is thin. Corrective measures include placing the implant under the muscle (if it was previously over the muscle), replacing a textured implant with one that is smooth, or adding a layer of ADM between the implant and the skin. Saline implants more frequently show ripples and wrinkles, and for that reason, they are routinely overfilled to decrease the likelihood of this occurring, but this also makes the implant more firm. (Each implant has a range for overfilling set by the manufacturer; exceeding these limits can affect the implant durability and may void the warranty.)

Gel bleed. Despite the cohesiveness of silicone gel, droplets of oil can leak through the implant shell into the surrounding capsule of scar tissue. This *gel bleed* can occur in all silicone implants. It may occur less frequently in highly cohesive gel devices, although no long-term evidence supports or refutes this belief. However, an interesting study involving pigs showed that cohesive silicone implants bled as much as the two previous generations of silicone implants.[8] Gel bleed is concerning because it can incite an inflammatory response in the scar capsule, which may lead to capsular contracture. It can also migrate to the lymph nodes or other areas of the body, causing hard lumps that require professional evaluation. FDA investigations have shown no evidence of harm from silicone exposure, and a 1999 Institute of Medicine report determined that human exposure to silicones, even at high doses, doesn't cause serious or long-term health problems. Silicone is manufactured by combining certain chemical substances with silicon, the second-most common natural chemical element on the planet. Silicon is ubiquitous in the environment; we're all exposed to it as a part of modern life. It's used in thousands of everyday products, including cosmetics, non-stick cookware, and even antacids. It's commonly found in small amounts in the body, including in breast milk, even in individuals who don't have silicone implants.

Cosmetic issues. While any reconstructive surgery has the potential for cosmetic problems, some are unique to breast implants. Cosmetic issues can generally be improved or resolved, although additional surgery may be required.

- *Asymmetry* can often be corrected by injecting liposuctioned fat into the breast or by replacing the implants. After unilateral reconstruction, it can be difficult to match your natural breast without additional surgery, because implants can't be shaped and sculpted like living tissue. You may become more asymmetrical over time, because your implanted breast won't droop or reflect weight changes as your natural breast does.

- *Malpositioned* implants move too far up, down, or to the sides of the pocket. If the breast skin stretches too much, implants can "bottom out," drifting below the inframammary crease. Patches of ADM can be added beneath or along the sides of the implant to improve its positioning and keep it where it belongs.

- Implant movement can be excessive if the pocket is too large. One method of repair is to return to the operating room to remove the implant and surgically reduce the pocket. If implant movement is minimal, an easier fix is to place a small ADM graft around the implant, reducing the space between the implant and the pocket.

- The weight of the implant may cause *extrusion*, so that it breaks through the skin, particularly in women who smoke or have thin or radiated skin. When this occurs, the implant must be removed and the skin allowed to heal before a new implant can be placed.

- *Symmastia* occurs when the sub-muscular pockets are too close together and eliminate the natural space between the breasts—the breasts appear as though they're joined in the middle, creating a condition sometimes called "uniboob." This happens when too much of the muscle is cut when the pockets are formed or using implants that are too big or too wide. Repair involves reducing the pocket size or reinforcing the inside borders of the pockets with ADM to hold the implants in proper position.

- Insufficient cleavage can be improved with fat grafting or by using larger or wider implants.

Removing or replacing your implant. Like washing machines, tires, and other manufactured products, implants eventually wear out. They have no finite shelf life, and there's no way to predict how long yours will last, although improvements continue to be made and newer implants, especially those with cohesive silicone gel, are expected to last longer. Some women have their implants for 10 to 20 years without complication, but most need to have them replaced at least once during their lifetime. According to the FDA, "The longer a woman has silicone gel–filled breast implants, the more likely she is to experience local complications. As many as one in five primary augmentation patients and one in two primary reconstruction patients require device removal within 10 years of implantation."[9]

Unless complications occur, replacing an implant is not a particularly difficult procedure. The pocket is already there, so most of the work is done. Accessing the pocket through the mastectomy incision, excess scar tissue is removed, and the old implant is replaced with a new one. This is an *outpatient procedure* with minimal discomfort. If you decide not to replace your implants, you can opt for reconstruction with your own tissue. If you prefer to forgo any additional reconstruction, most of your breast skin will be removed and you'll have a slanting scar across your chest, as though you had a mastectomy without reconstruction.

No matter how simple it may be to replace an implant, the process can be emotionally disruptive: you're happily living your post-mastectomy life, and then you find that you need more doctor visits and additional surgery to repair a problem with your new breast. Some women say it's like reliving their reconstruction all over again. Other women consider replacement surgery a price they're willing to pay. Either way, it's an important consideration when deciding which reconstructive technique is best for you.

> *I don't mind if the implant must be exchanged in the future. I consider it required maintenance, like getting my car serviced. I can take time to do that if I need to. Besides, maybe they'll have something better and I can trade up to a better model!* —Belle

Implant warranties. Before your initial surgery, your doctor or a member of the office staff should provide you with a copy of the manufacturer's implant warranty and explain its terms. (You can also read the warranty terms online at the manufacturer's website.) Once your implants are in place, be sure you have your implant ID card, which lists your implant's manufacturer, type, size, and serial numbers, before you leave the hospital. You'll need this information to register your warranty.

CHAPTER SEVEN

The Expander Experience

I was excited to watch the "growing" process unfold each week. —LENORE

Although tissue expansion can be tedious, it's an amazing process. Two helpful step-by-step photo journals of the procedure are "Mastectomy & Breast Reconstruction: Expanders to Implants" (http://lianne-brca2.livejournal .com) and "Myself: Together Again" (www.myselftogetheragain.org).

Getting Your Fill

When your mastectomy incision has healed sufficiently, usually in three or four weeks, you'll begin regular visits to your plastic surgeon's office to gradually fill your expanders. (If you develop a post-mastectomy infection or other complication, your fills may be delayed until the problem is resolved.) Your surgeon will inject 50 to 100 cc (about 3.5 to 7 tablespoons) or more of sterile saline through a valve on the expander (figure 7.1)—you may be able to feel the valve when you run your fingers over your breast skin. (If you need post-mastectomy radiation, request expanders with plastic ports; when radiated, metal ports can damage the skin.) You probably won't feel the needle, because your breast will be numb, although some women say that it feels like a bee sting. You'll feel pressure as your new breast mound "grows" to accommodate the saline. Every week or two, you'll return to repeat the process, which takes only a few minutes. With each fill, your breast mound grows a bit more and the inframammary fold forms under your breast. During your last appointment, your expander will be somewhat overfilled. This ensures that you'll have sufficient skin to cover your implant and enough space so that it will sit low in the pocket with a more natural droop, instead of unnaturally high on your chest. Most women are completely filled in six to eight weeks. Your own interval may

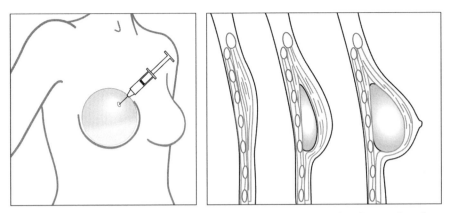

FIGURE 7.1. Adding saline to the tissue expander (*left*) gradually stretches the muscle and surrounding skin, until the flat mastectomy site slowly grows into a fully formed breast mound (*right*).

TABLE 7.1. Sample intervals for tissue expansion

Volume added at biweekly fill (cc)*	Total volume of implant (cc)			
	6 weeks	8 weeks	10 weeks	12 weeks
60	240	300	360	420
100	360	460	560	660
140	480	620	—	—

*Assumptions: 60 cc added at initial surgery; each fill adds equal amount of saline.

be shorter or longer, depending on the elasticity and the fragility of your skin, how much it needs to stretch to accommodate the implant, and how well you tolerate the process. If your surgeon recommends a more conservative approach, the process will take longer (table 7.1). Expanding radiated skin can be especially challenging and must proceed slowly (it can add several weeks to the expansion timeline), especially when the skin is very thin or the tissue is scarred and thickened. Expanding radiated skin sometimes works. Sometimes it doesn't. It helps to have a plastic surgeon with a good deal of experience working with radiated skin and tissue.

Using an acellular dermal matrix can shorten the expansion interval; more saline can be added during the initial operation and in subsequent fills, completing your expansion sooner. If you have chemotherapy treatments during expansion, talk to your doctor about the best time to have your fills. It may be helpful to have them a day or two before your chemo, when your resistance to infection is strongest.

AeroForm expanders (www.Airxpanders.com) offer a do-it-yourself approach to tissue expansion. You use a wireless remote control to release up to 30 cc of carbon dioxide per day (three doses of 10 cc each) from a small reservoir within the contoured expander, in your own home and at your own pace. You control when, where, and how much you're expanded, with less discomfort and without injections or office visits. (Your surgeon may want to see you once or twice during the fill process to make sure you're progressing adequately.) It also shortens the expansion interval: during an FDA pre-approval clinical trial, women who used AeroForm expanders reached their targeted volume in an average of 18.2 days, compared to an average of 57.4 days for women who randomly received traditional expanders.[1]

Minimizing Your Discomfort

Expanders are built for function, to create room for your implants, and not so much for comfort or form. Some women sail through the process with minimal discomfort, whereas others find it annoying, stressful, and uncomfortable. The lower portion of your chest where the muscles attach to the ribs will feel tight. Your chest may feel heavy or tender, particularly if your breast was previously radiated. It will feel fuller and tighter each time more saline is added, but in most cases, this subsides within a few hours. It's a bit like having dental braces—just when you get used to them, the dentist tightens them, and they're uncomfortable all over again. Your pectoral muscles may contract or spasm as they stretch between fills. One day, the muscles will relax, and you'll feel much better. In the meantime, try the following tips to relieve your discomfort:

- Pain medication isn't usually required during fills. However, if the process is too uncomfortable, talk to your surgeon about taking acetaminophen (Tylenol) or an over-the-counter anti-inflammatory immediately before or after more saline is added. If that doesn't do the trick, ask your surgeon to prescribe a muscle relaxant, anti-inflammatory, or pain medication.

- Apply a cold pack (ice cubes or frozen peas wrapped in a towel) for up to 20 minutes at a time for temporary relief.

- Try gentle self-massage along the front and side of your rib cage to relax your muscles. Or ask your surgeon for a referral to a physical therapist, who can massage and relax the connective tissues in your chest.

- Exercise is beneficial during expansion, as long as it doesn't involve high-impact activities such as aerobics, jogging, or swimming until your surgeon gives you the okay. Slowly and gently move your arms to stretch your pectoral muscles. Avoid lifting weights or other activities that increase or strengthen your pectoralis muscles, so it won't become more difficult to stretch them.

- If your expansion is unbearable, ask your surgeon to remove some saline from your expander, allow more time between fills, or add less saline each time. You'll be eager to be done with the process, but take time to listen to your body. It will be worth it in the long run. Or consider having Botox injected directly into the chest muscle: small trials show that women who had injections suffered fewer muscle spasms, needed less pain medication during expansion, and tolerated larger fills.[2]

I had an amazing experience with tissue expanders without any real complications. The pain was brutal at times but was mostly relieved with medication. Staying on top of pain meds, resting when needed, and using muscle relaxants made it very doable. I was excited to watch the "growing" process unfold each week. I was truly in awe after each fill, despite the tightness that occurred a few hours later and continued through the evening. However, the next day I felt well again. I resumed gym activities after my first expansion, and my exchange surgery went off without a hitch. I returned to full-time work five weeks after my mastectomy. Tissue expanders are not for everyone, but they can be a positive experience for those who go into the procedure knowing what to expect. —Lenore

Once I scheduled my mastectomy and tissue expander surgery, I had plenty of time to worry. I spent hours on the Internet reading about it. I also

watched videos about women going through expansion, and they made the fills seem so painful! The first time I had a fill I was pretty nervous. Honestly, I felt the first contact the needle had with my skin, almost like a bug bite. After that, the only discomfort was at the end, when the muscle and skin stretched. I took Tylenol before and after the fill. That really works! Other than that, I went about my day after the fill, and even went to the gym. By nighttime, the discomfort was completely gone, and I would forget all about it until my next appointment.   —Michelle

My doctor began filling my expanders with 120 cc every seven days. I was very uncomfortable for two or three days afterward. It felt like a metal band was crushing my ribs. I finally asked him to put in only 60 cc at a time. My expansion took longer, but it was more tolerable.   —Lin

Living in Limbo

After surgery to place your tissue expanders, you'll leave the hospital with a surgical bra. When your doctor clears you to wear your own bra, be sure it fit wells and doesn't compress the expander. Avoid underwire bras, which can put too much pressure on the inframammary fold of your new breast, until your surgeon says you've healed sufficiently to wear them again.

Dressing during the expansion process can be a challenge. During unilateral expansion, your growing breast mound may not be the same size or shape as your healthy breast, and it may sit higher on your chest, so it may be difficult to find a bra that fits both. A small prosthesis in your bra may help to correct an imbalance in your shape. You can also wear a padded mastectomy bra while your new breast is being expanded. As your breast mound grows, remove some of the stuffing from that side of the bra to give yourself a more symmetrical look.

The expansion process may seem endless, and you may become impatient with the tightness and cosmetic annoyances, but there is light at the end of the tunnel. Don't be disheartened with your asymmetry. Hang in there if you feel lopsided or misshapen, or if your reconstructed breasts are flatter or rounder than you expected. If you develop "neck cleavage," where the expander rides high up on the chest, your surgeon can force it into a lower position with an elastic bandage. Don't be overly concerned with incisions that seem uneven or puckered; they can be improved during your exchange surgery. Remember, you're a work in progress. Expanders are temporary. Your discomfort is temporary. And this isn't the way your finished breast will look or feel. Keep the end result in mind, and in a few weeks, your expansion will be complete.

> *It was very difficult initially for me to look at the bruising and the flatter, misshapen appearance of my breasts, but my husband, and the doctor and his staff were very encouraging and gave me confidence and peace of mind that this phase was only temporary. Once my incisions were healed, I was fitted for breast forms and mastectomy bras by a certified fitter. The bras and forms were covered by my insurance, and I was able to wear them under my clothes while my expansion was being completed. I didn't need the forms for very long, but it was a blessing to have the option to have a formed breast silhouette on some occasions with certain clothes.* —Cara

Exchange Surgery

Surgeons have different ideas about how long expanders should stay in before replacing them with implants. Some like to rush the process along. Others prefer to be more cautious, particularly if your skin will benefit from taking it slow. For most women, exchange surgery can be performed four to six weeks after the last fill, when the pectoral muscles have stretched sufficiently and the expanders have settled into the pocket. Some women keep their expanders for months before replacing them with implants. You may need to wait a while longer if your surgeon wants to give your radiated skin more time to heal or if your schedule causes a delay.

Some expanders are adjustable, with an outer layer of silicone and an inner chamber that is inflated with saline. These combined expander-implants do double duty—saline can be added or removed to fine-tune your breast size during the six months after the implant is fully expanded. Then the fill valve is removed, triggering the expander to seal itself. The expander becomes the implant, eliminating the need for exchange surgery.

Exchange surgery is an outpatient procedure. Once you're asleep, the surgeon reopens your mastectomy scar and removes the expander. He may also remove scar tissue from the pocket, which will soften the overall appearance of your breast. Your new implant goes into the pocket and is adjusted to match the position of your opposite breast. The incision is closed, and a surgical bra is put in place to discourage swelling.

Compared with your initial operation, exchange surgery is a snap. The procedure takes about an hour for each breast. You'll notice the difference as soon as you wake up: most if not all of the tightness will be gone, and your implants will feel vastly more comfortable than your expanders. You should be back to your normal routine in just a few days. At your post-op appointment in about a week, your surgeon will remove the hospital dressing, and for the first time, you'll get a look at your new breasts. They'll be a big improvement over the expanders, but they're still not the final product. Over the next few weeks, the swelling will subside, and your implants will drop to a more normal position. They'll continue to settle and become softer over the next several months.

I was amazed to have hardly any swelling or bruising after my mastectomy, and I did have cleavage from the expanders! At first, they gave me a flat bulk, like a bodybuilder. My new breasts looked okay when I looked down, but there wasn't much there from a side view. I was so upset. Even though the expanders were better than no breasts at all; they were nothing like the breasts I had seen in my surgeon's patient photos. In hindsight, I should have listened to my surgeon, who said my implants would be very different. Of course, he was right. My implants are so much better than the expanders, and they continue to improve.   —Carole

Potential Problems

Most women don't have serious problems with tissue expanders, but complications can occur. Expanders aren't recommended if you have poor circulation in your chest, a history of poor wound healing, or an infection anywhere in your body. Delayed healing after mastectomy, insufficient blood flow to the skin, or other problems may also postpone or preclude using expanders. Tobacco use, secondhand smoke, or other possible causes of blood flow problems may compromise circulation after mastectomy. If the breast skin dies, the expanders must be removed.

Expanders can rupture if they're damaged or compressed excessively or if the valve is defective. Be protective of your chest during your expansion. A fall against furniture or an unintended blow to your chest can cause a rupture so that the expander leaks saline, loses volume and shape, and needs to be removed to prevent infection. It's a frustrating setback, but a new expander can be put in, and your reconstruction can continue. Replacement may also be required when infection develops or significant capsular contracture occurs.

CHAPTER EIGHT

Tummy Tuck Flaps

*Honestly, my TRAM hurt like hell . . . Now I'm just as
excited about my flat stomach as I am my new breast.*

—MONIQUE

Not so long ago, the goal of breast reconstruction was simply to give a
woman something more permanent than a prosthesis to fill her bra. *Tissue flap* reconstruction (also called *autologous reconstruction*) creates entirely new possibilities by replacing lost breast tissue with your own living
tissue, recreating a soft breast that becomes an integral part of your body.
Flap reconstruction is used as a primary method of recreating the breasts
or to replace failed implant reconstruction. (The opposite—using expanders or implants to replace a failed flap reconstruction—can also be done.)

Tissue Flap Basics

Flap procedures transfer a segment of living tissue, including its blood
supply, up to the chest, where it is shaped into a breast. Compared with
implant procedures, reconstruction with your own tissue is a longer
operation and is initially more intense, but the start-to-finish interval is
shorter than for traditional implant reconstruction with expansion (figure 8.1). As scars fade and tissue softens, the new breast improves over
time. Flap surgery can be done only once from a particular *donor site*; if
you need a future reconstruction, a tissue flap from a different area of your
body or a breast implant must be used.

Look at the human anatomy and you'll see three distinct layers of tissue over the body's organs: skin on top, fat in the middle, and muscle
underneath, with blood vessels running through all three layers. The distinction among various tissue flap techniques, aside from the location of
the donor site, is how these blood vessels are included in the flap. This is

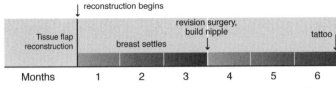

FIGURE 8.1. Tissue flap reconstruction timeline. Intervals may differ, depending on breast cancer treatment, preference of patient and surgeon, and complications that may delay completion.

the most critical part of flap reconstruction, because once in place in the chest, the transferred tissue needs a robust blood supply to deliver oxygen and nutrients to the new breast. Without it, some or all of the flap will die. Three types of flap procedures are used, each accessing the needed blood vessels in a different way and requiring different surgical skills. Not all plastic surgeons are trained to perform autologous reconstruction, and not all surgeons who perform this type of reconstruction are qualified to do all tissue flap variations.

Attached (pedicled) flaps use skin, fat, and muscle. A flap of skin and fat is cut away but left attached to one end of the muscle and tunneled under the skin to the chest. The other end of the muscle remains in place. The biggest drawback of an attached flap is that it sacrifices a perfectly healthy muscle, which isn't necessary to build the breast but is taken only for the blood supply that runs through it. Attached flaps are the original method of natural tissue reconstruction; they were developed at a time when it was necessary to sacrifice the muscle for the blood supply within.

The advent of *microsurgery* revolutionized the way blood supply to the flap is harvested, so that the muscle is preserved. Using high-powered magnifying equipment and delicate instruments, specially trained *microsurgeons* can disconnect tiny blood vessels in the flap and reconnect them to blood vessels in the chest or underarm with sutures that are thinner than human hair, eliminating the need to sacrifice an entire muscle. (A small piece of rib cartilage is removed to gain better access to the internal artery in the chest, particularly in women with narrow or small chests.) Microsurgery allows less invasive procedures and less damage at the donor site, which translates into easier recovery and fewer complications. *Free flaps* are microsurgical procedures. They are complete transplants of tissue from the donor site to the chest. A free flap includes just a portion of muscle—the amount removed varies between surgeons—that surrounds the necessary blood supply. Detaching and reconnecting vessels temporarily interrupts the supply of blood. This isn't a problem if the reconnection is completed within 30 to 45 minutes.

Perforator flaps require the most advanced microsurgical techniques. Named for the small arteries that run through muscle, these flaps use only skin and fat, preserving all of the muscle at the donor site. A preoperative *CT angiogram,* a type of scan that views the underlying blood vessels, shows whether they are intact and undamaged. This is particularly important for women who have had previous abdominal surgery. Rather than removing any portion of a muscle to obtain the blood vessels inside, this procedure involves carefully extracting the *perforating artery* from the underlying muscle and moving it along with the flap of skin and fat to the mastectomy site, where it is reconnected in the chest. This requires the most microsurgical skill, experience, and technical savvy of all reconstruction procedures. Perforator flap reconstruction is complex and lengthy microsurgery, but compared with attached flap procedures, it's a less debilitating operation with a shorter hospital stay and quicker recovery.

ADVANTAGES OF TISSUE FLAP RECONSTRUCTION

- *It creates a breast with a natural feel, look, and movement.*
- *It offers a better chance of regaining sensation.*
- *No tissue expansion is required.*
- *It avoids the complications related to implants.*
- *It is less likely than implants to be compromised by previous radiation.*
- *Matching the normal droop of the opposite breast is easier (after unilateral mastectomy).*
- *It improves contour at the donor site, particularly the hips, thighs, and abdomen.*
- *It lasts a lifetime.*

DISADVANTAGES OF TISSUE FLAP RECONSTRUCTION

- *It scars an otherwise healthy part of the body.*
- *Some procedures sacrifice muscle.*
- *Surgery and recovery are longer and more intense than for implant procedures.*

- *It usually requires a second-stage revision surgery.*
- *The area around the donor site incision may remain permanently numb.*
- *Future weight loss or gain may affect the volume of the new breast.*
- *Fewer surgeons are qualified and experienced in these techniques.*

Once the breast has settled into position (at least three months after reconstruction), a return trip to the operating room for revision procedures can improve shape and symmetry. Fat liposuctioned from your hips, thighs, or other locations can be injected into the new breast to fill sunken areas, add moderate volume, and improve contour (chapter 10). Your incision scar can be revised, if necessary. This is the stage when new nipples are created. If you had unilateral reconstruction, your opposite breast can be modified at this stage for better symmetry with your reconstructed breast.

The length of revision surgery depends on how much work needs to be done. Although not all problems can be resolved, they can usually be improved. In the hands of a competent plastic surgeon, revision surgery can make subtle changes that improve the look of your new breasts.

Borrowing from the Abdomen

The abdomen is the most common donor site for flap reconstruction, providing a two-for-one benefit—the same tissue normally removed and discarded after a tummy tuck is used to create the new breast mound. You come out of reconstructive surgery with new breasts *and* a flatter belly, thereby slimming your overall body contour. Abdominal tissue is a good choice for reconstruction because it has skin tone and texture similar to breast tissue.

Beneath the abdominal skin and fat are the long, flat rectus abdominis ("six-pack") muscles. You have two: one on the left and one on the right, both extending from the fifth, sixth, and seventh ribs to the pubic bone. These are the sit-up muscles that support the abdominal wall, help you to bend and flex at the waist, and keep your abdominal organs in place. Each muscle has two sources of blood, the superior artery and veins at the top and the inferior artery and veins near the groin.

Abdominal flap procedures begin with a hip-to-hip elliptical incision above the navel and almost to the pubic bone, similar to the placement of a horizontal cesarean incision. The resulting scar will be covered by most bathing suits and underwear. Your belly button may look different after your surgery. During the operation, it's freed from the surrounding skin but remains attached to the abdominal wall. When the flap has been removed and the edges of the incision are pulled together, a new hole is made and the belly button is pulled through and sutured in place with tiny stitches.

Unless you have an abundance of excess abdominal tissue, you might wonder whether you should try to gain weight before your reconstruction, especially if you don't have enough abdominal tissue to make a breast of the size you'd like. Considering the health problems associated with obesity, many experts consider deliberate weight gain to be inadvisable. On the contrary, you should strive to be in the best shape you can before your procedure, to better facilitate your recovery. Also, it's difficult to target weight gain exclusively to the tummy or other specific place on the body. And even though a part of your tummy is now in your breast, it will continue to respond to diet and exercise, reflecting overall weight losses and gains as though it were still in its original location.

TRAM Flap Procedures

Introduced in the 1980s, the *transverse rectus abdominis myocutaneous (TRAM) flap* was the first abdominal flap technique developed for breast reconstruction. It was a significant step forward, because it gave women an alternative to implant reconstruction and an opportunity to have new breasts of their own living tissue. While *attached (pedicled) TRAM* is no longer the most advanced flap reconstruction, it's still the most common, because it doesn't require microsurgical training or skill, and it is widely available. Attached TRAM is not the best option for women who have compromised circulation due to smoking, diabetes, obesity, or other conditions, or who have had previous abdominal surgery.

How an attached TRAM is done. The rectus abdominis muscle opposite the missing breast is used for unilateral reconstruction; both muscles are used for bilateral reconstruction. A flap of skin, fat, and underlying muscle is cut away from the lower abdomen; the upper end of the muscle

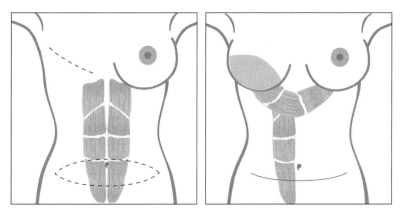

FIGURE 8.2. In the attached TRAM procedure, a flap of skin and fat remains attached to one end of the rectus abdominis muscle, and is tunneled under the skin to the chest. The opposite end of the muscle remains in place.

remains attached in its original position above the rib cage to provide blood to the flap (figure 8.2). The flap is then tunneled under the skin to the mastectomy site. The upper portion is sutured into position to provide fullness at the top of the new breast, while the lower edge of the flap is folded under, shaped to match the size and contour of the opposite breast, and sutured in place. The edges of the abdominal incision are pulled together and closed.

Recovery. Attached TRAM surgery is serious business. You're recovering from not one but two significant operations and the loss of one or both major abdominal muscles. It's the most difficult recovery of any breast reconstruction procedure.

It's amazing how many movements involve the abdominal muscles; that's something you'll discover after a TRAM operation. Lifting, bending, and other movements we take for granted will be difficult until your incision heals. You'll need help getting in and out of bed, especially if both muscles were removed. Your abdomen will feel very sore and very tight, and you'll feel a pulling sensation that may last for several months but slowly improves. Because it will be difficult to stand straight, you'll want to slouch until you recover, but it's very important that you move and walk, gradually standing straighter as your incision heals. You may need four to six weeks until you can begin gentle stretching; you'll gradually begin more vigorous movement and should be back to most routine activities within two months, although women sometimes require additional time to heal. You may feel tired for several more weeks as your energy level slowly returns and may need more time before resuming more strenuous movements and activities. For the first two or three months after your surgery, your reconstructed breast will be swollen and look fuller than its final size. Over several months, as the swelling subsides and the muscle thins from lack of exercise, your new breast will assume its final shape. It may take up to a year for the underlying tissues to heal completely.

Most women have no long-term ill effects from an attached TRAM, but without the support of the rectus muscle, it's not possible to do sit-ups or get in and out of bed without first rolling to the side. Removing the six-pack muscles and the *fascia* (the fibrous tissue covering the muscles) weakens the abdominal wall, which limits strength and range of motion. A *hernia*, a bulge under the skin caused by the intestines poking through the muscle, may also occur as a result of the weakened abdominal wall. It's a painful condition that may require surgery to repair the muscle. The risk of hernia is greater if you're obese. Many surgeons reinforce the abdomen with surgical mesh after removing the muscle. If you are planning to have this type of reconstruction, ask your surgeon how he will address the residual abdominal weakness. A different type of bulge may develop five or six months after the operation as a result of tunneling tissue under the skin; this usually recedes as the muscle atrophies and thins. You may need physical therapy to strengthen your remaining core muscles and improve posture and mobility.

Pregnancy after TRAM. After a TRAM procedure, especially bilateral TRAM, it's questionable whether the weakened abdominal walls can withstand the stress of pregnancy. There is little evidence or documented statistics one way or the other, and traditionally, many experts advise against future pregnancies for TRAM patients. A 2015 analysis of published literature on the subject identified 18 women who became pregnant between 3 and 46 months after unilateral or bilateral TRAM—two were unknowingly pregnant at the time of their TRAM procedures. All 20 women had normal full-term pregnancies; 15 had vaginal deliveries and 5 had a cesarean section.[1] Most women had no significant complications. One developed an abdominal hernia, three had bulges in the abdominal wall, and one woman's scar became hypertrophic (it stretched beyond the level of the TRAM incision). Some of the women had abdominal mesh in place following their TRAM procedures; it's unclear whether all of them did. Although this seems to imply that pregnancy is safe after attached TRAM, these are individual cases, without sufficient evidence to identify potential risks, to suggest how long TRAM patients should wait before becoming pregnant, or to clarify which women are candidates for pregnancy without significant complications. If you hope for a future pregnancy, be sure to discuss this with your obstetrician/gynecologist to determine whether reconstruction with a muscle-sparing procedure or implants may be a wiser choice.

When I woke up from my TRAM operation, I felt as though I had been hit by a bus. The first week or so, I thought I'd made a terrible mistake. I had medication and the pain improved a little each day, but the first week was awful. I couldn't stand or sit up straight for almost three weeks. —Teri

Honestly, my TRAM hurt like hell. I spent a lot of the day crying and just stayed on medication until I got better. Now I'm just as excited about my flat stomach as I am my new breast. For the first time in my life, I'm a babe! I'm wearing clothes I never would have worn before my surgery. —Monique

My cousin had a TRAM flap the year before I did. I was about 20 pounds overweight; she was in good shape. Her first seven or eight days were painful, and then she steadily improved. I had quite a bit of pain for three weeks. —Carrie

Variations on the TRAM flap. *Free TRAM* reconstruction uses the same tissue as the attached TRAM procedure but removes only a portion of the muscle surrounding the blood supply. Instead of tunneling the flap under the skin, it is cut away from the abdominal muscle and transferred to the chest. Severing the blood vessels from the abdomen and reattaching them in the chest requires microsurgical skills and makes for a longer, more complex operation than an attached TRAM procedure; yet, it also provides advantages: a more reliable blood supply that translates to less risk of necrosis and other healing problems. Compared to an attached TRAM, this is a better option for women whose circulation is compromised. Transplanting the flap to the mastectomy site also eliminates bulges near the rib cage that often result from tunneling muscle under the skin and reduces the risk of hernia. Although the muscle remains in the abdomen, it is cut across its width to remove the small amount included in the flap. So even though most of the muscle is left in place, much of its function is destroyed. The amount of muscle that is removed varies between surgeons; more experienced surgeons can perform the procedure while removing less muscle. Recovery is similar but somewhat less intense than what is experienced with an attached TRAM.

A *muscle-sparing TRAM* removes a very small amount of muscle, often described as the size of a postage stamp. Because most muscle integrity, strength, and function are preserved, you get the benefits of a free TRAM procedure without most of the disadvantages. Recovery is shorter and less painful, and the risk of hernia is reduced (surgical mesh isn't usually needed).

DIEP and SIEA Flaps

Why sacrifice a perfectly good muscle if you don't need to? That's the philosophy behind the *deep inferior epigastric perforator (DIEP) flap*, the most advanced breast reconstruction procedure with abdominal tissue (figure 8.3). DIEP flap reconstruction uses only what is needed for the new breast: the same fat and skin as other TRAM procedures but none of the muscle. Complication rates tend to be lower than TRAM procedures (table 8.1).[2] You aren't a candidate for DIEP if you've already had a TRAM procedure or a full tummy tuck. A prior cesarean delivery, hysterectomy, liposuction, tubal ligation, or gallbladder surgery doesn't usually eliminate DIEP as a possible reconstructive method, as long as you have enough tissue and the perforator artery hasn't been damaged. A previous appendectomy may be a problem if it damaged the blood vessels for the flap. The more abdominal surgeries you've previously had, the higher the risk of bulging or hernia and the trickier it is to perform a DIEP with a successful outcome.

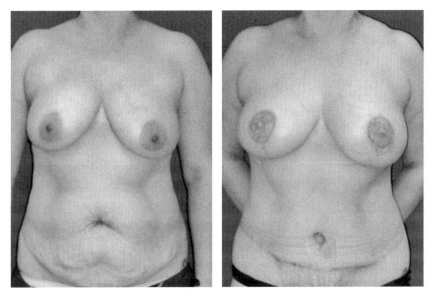

FIGURE 8.3. Before (*left*) and after (*right*) immediate bilateral DIEP reconstruction, with later nipple reconstruction and tattoos. Images provided by Dr. Minas Chrysopoulo, PRMA Center for Advanced Breast Reconstruction.

TABLE 8.1. Percentage of complications with abdominal tissue flaps

	Attached TRAM	Free TRAM	Muscle-sparing TRAM	DIEP
Hernia/bulging	16.6	5.6	8.2	4.2
Infection	15.7	9.7	7.2	6.3
Necrosis	25.3	16.7	15.0	16.3
Partial flap loss	8.9	7.6	4.8	4.0
Total flap	1.2	2.1	1.4	1.6

How it's done. Few surgeons have the meticulous skill and experience needed to perform this complex operation successfully with minimal impact to the rectus abdominis muscle. The flap of skin and fat is separated from the muscle and lifted up, exposing the inferior perforator arteries that branch out from a main artery and run through the muscle (figure 8.4). Unlike a free TRAM or muscle-sparing TRAM, the rectus muscle isn't cut. A small incision is made into the fascia, and the blood vessels are carefully teased away from the muscle. The surgeon must take care to

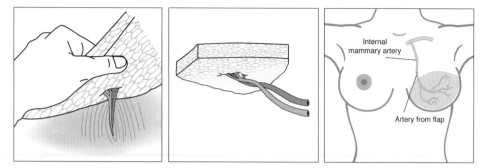

FIGURE 8.4. In perforator flap reconstruction, the flap of fat and skin is lifted away from the muscle (*left*). The perforator artery and veins are detached from the muscle (*center*), and are reconnected to blood vessels in the chest (*right*).

preserve the adjacent motor nerves; if they're damaged or severed, some abdominal muscle function could be lost. If the perforator artery is tangled with scar tissue (perhaps from a previous cesarean section) or a cluster of muscle fibers, a very small incision may be required. But typically, a DIEP procedure doesn't involve an incision in the muscle. The entire flap with its blood supply is then moved up to the mastectomy site, the perforator artery is reconnected in the chest, and the abdominal tissue is shaped into a breast. The incision is pulled together and closed. (A *periumbilical perforator* [PUP] *flap* uses the same tissue but includes a perforator artery that is closer to the navel.) From the outside, there's little visible difference between a breast created with a TRAM or a DIEP. The difference, which is significant, is all on the inside—you leave the hospital with new breasts and fully functional abdominal muscles.

Variations on the DIEP flap. DIEP flap techniques can be modified for thin women who want a flap reconstruction but don't have quite enough fatty tissue. In an *extended DIEP*, the standard hip-to-hip incision is lengthened to include both abdominal and hip fat for additional volume. The *stacked DIEP* (also called a *double DIEP*) combines flaps to provide enough volume for a unilateral reconstruction; the entire abdominal flap is harvested in one segment and folded over to create the breast or both sides are harvested separately and stacked one on top of the other. The result is a new breast that has more fullness and projection than a breast made from a single smaller flap.

In a small percentage of women (an estimated 15 percent), the *superficial inferior epigastric artery (SIEA)* is an acceptable alternative blood supply for the flap (figure 8.5). Although the surgery and cosmetic result of a SIEA flap are essentially the same as those for a DIEP flap, SIEA blood vessels are found in the fatty tissue just beneath the skin. Recovery is improved, because the abdominal muscle is not only spared but undisturbed. In most women, the superficial blood vessels are too small to support the flap; they've already been cut during a previous cesarean delivery, tummy tuck, or hysterectomy; or they don't exist. The existence and adequacy of the SIEA blood supply is assessed in the operating room.

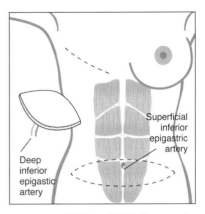

FIGURE 8.5. DIEP and SIEA flaps use fat and skin but no muscle.

When surgeons discover during surgery that the perforator arteries are damaged or too small to adequately supply the flap, a free TRAM can be performed instead. Mapping the blood vessels to determine the exact location and caliber of the blood flow before surgery saves time in the operating room. Blood vessels can be evaluated with a handheld *Doppler* to evaluate blood flow in perforators during your consultation appointment or with color Doppler ultrasound, a special MRI, or a CT angiogram that views the underlying blood vessels to determine whether they are intact and undamaged. This is particularly important for women who have had previous abdominal surgery. Similar internal mapping can be performed in the operating room before an incision is made, by using a special dye and imaging technology to assess the perforator vessels as they travel through the tissue.

Finding a DIEP/SIEA surgeon. Because most reconstructive surgeons aren't trained in microsurgical breast reconstruction, the most important factor in any perforator flap reconstruction is choosing a microsurgeon who routinely performs these procedures. Operating intervals and success rates vary among individual surgeons. Those who routinely perform DIEP reconstruction are likely to complete the procedure in less time than those

TABLE 8.2. Intervals for abdominal flap reconstruction and recovery

Flap type	Surgery and hospital stay	Most routine activities resumed*
Attached TRAM	4–6 hours; 3–5 days in hospital	6–8 weeks
Free TRAM	6–8 hours; 4–5 days in hospital	4–6 weeks
DIEP or SIEA	5–8 hours; 4–5 days in hospital	4–6 weeks

Note: Reflects bilateral reconstruction without complications. Surgical expertise and individual healing affect recovery times.
*Additional time needed to regain full strength and mobility or return to strenuous activity.

who do not, resolve problems when they occur, and their success rates may be higher.

The only person qualified to assess whether you have enough tissue for a DIEP reconstruction is a plastic surgeon who routinely performs the procedure. If a surgeon who performs only implant reconstruction, TRAM, or other non-DIEP procedures suggests you don't have enough belly fat for a DIEP, an experienced DIEP surgeon may disagree. Likewise, if a surgeon says he needs to take only a small portion of muscle for a DIEP, he's actually talking about a free TRAM or muscle-sparing TRAM. You're lucky if you have an accomplished DIEP surgeon in a teaching university or private practice nearby (check the list of microsurgeons at www .breastrecon.com). Many women are willing to travel out of state or across the country for their microsurgical reconstruction.

Recovery. Patients have less pain and get back to their normal activities sooner after DIEP than other abdominal flap procedures; it's still major surgery that requires recuperation (table 8.2). Although you'll take short walks every day in the hospital, it will probably take another 10 days to 2 weeks until you can stand upright and walk normally. Each day you'll feel progressively better and less fatigued. Many women return to work in about 4 weeks, while some require additional recovery. Strenuous exercise should be avoided for at least a couple of months after your surgery. By 6 weeks (and maybe sooner), you'll be able to drive and resume your routine activities. As for all surgeries, recovery varies from patient to patient.

I play a lot of tennis, so I was in pretty good shape before my surgery. I wanted to get back on the court as soon as possible, so I had a DIEP operation. I was out of it for several days, although I recovered well and was back to most of my routine in about a month. —Casey

When I decided to have DIEP reconstruction, I met with many surgeons. When my hometown doctors said I didn't have enough donor tissue, I traveled across most of the country for my surgeries and have never looked back—I returned home with two beautiful D-cup breasts. The experience was surreal, but I chose the most competent and caring doctors I have ever met in my entire life. I now live in Israel, and when my doctors here see my results, they are blown away. My recovery was uneventful; only some spitting stitches and hypertrophic scars. I was walking around by the third week and was [walking] up to four miles in another week or two. I drove by week six and returned to my desk job the following week. Five years later, I live a normal life. I see my scars but I do not regret my surgery one bit. —Debbie

Potential Problems

Although flap reconstruction with your own tissue doesn't involve the potential problems associated with breast implants, complications can occur. The success of reconstruction with a flap relies primarily on the strength of the blood supply. If the flap has adequate blood, it survives. If it doesn't, a portion of it may die off, become unusually firm, and need to be removed. Or the entire flap may die and will need to be removed, but this is uncommon. An area of the new breast that appears much harder than the rest can also result from formation of scar tissue. Routine massage and the passage of time are often all that is needed for the tissue to soften.

Hernia is less likely after DIEP than with an attached TRAM, and no surgical mesh is required. Compared to younger women who have flap surgery, women who are age 65 or older have a higher risk of venous thromboembolism, a blood clot that forms in a deep vein or in the lung. The somewhat higher risk doesn't necessarily preclude older women from having autologous breast reconstruction, but it does indicate that more precautions, such as the use of blood-thinning medications, should be taken with older women. If you're in this category, your physician can help you understand whether implant reconstruction is a better option for you. A small percentage of patients who take tamoxifen may also develop venous thromboembolism; your surgeon, with the consent of your oncologist, may advise you to stop taking it for a week or two before your operation.

Smoking or using any type of tobacco products makes you more susceptible to infection, seroma, hernia, and necrosis at both the mastectomy and donor sites. The risk of these problems can be reduced if you stop smoking for a month or more before your surgery. If you are obese, you have a greater chance of complications after a flap surgery, including seroma, infection, hernia, and partial or total flap loss.[3]

CHAPTER NINE

Other Flap Methods

I'm the world's biggest chicken when it comes to pain. I asked my doctor what method of reconstruction was the least painful.
—MARTA

If abdominal flap reconstruction isn't right for you, your breasts can be rebuilt with tissue from your back, buttocks, hips, or thighs. Although these procedures are used less often than implants or abdominal flaps, they produce very good reconstructive results.

Flaps from the Back

Originally developed to replace chest muscles after a radical mastectomy, *latissimus dorsi myocutaneous (lat) flap* reconstruction uses the flat, triangular back muscle that runs from the shoulder to the hip. (If you stand facing a wall and push against it, the latissimus dorsi is the muscle that enables that movement and facilitates twisting the body.) It's still a common method of reconstruction—it's performed about as often as TRAM procedures—and it's an alternative if you want a flap reconstruction but you don't have enough donor tissue elsewhere. Depending on where you live, it may be the only flap procedure available without traveling.

Because the muscle is thin and the flap tends to provide less fat than other donor sites, this method of reconstruction typically creates only a small to moderately sized breast and is often combined with an implant (with or without tissue expansion) for projection and volume. The horizontal donor site scar is easily covered by bras. The incision isn't as easily hidden when it's made diagonally, so if you choose this procedure, talk to your surgeon about the placement of your incision.

The thoracodorsal artery provides a reliable blood supply to the lat flap, which generally produces good results with few problems. For that reason, surgeons frequently recommend this reconstructive procedure for women who have already had radiation therapy to the chest. The flap brings healthy tissue to the radiated area and covers the implant completely, so rippling, wrinkling, and capsular contracture occur less often than with other implant procedures.[1] Because it is less likely to be impacted by delayed wound healing, the back flap is a good alternative for smokers, women who have diabetes, and women whose health precludes them from having longer, more invasive surgeries. If you have quite a bit of excess fat around the bra line on your back, a lat procedure can significantly improve that situation. It isn't a preferred option if you have circulatory problems, persistent pain, or weakness in your back or shoulder. Other methods of reconstruction may be better if you've had previous surgery in or adjacent to the underarm (which can disrupt blood flow to the flap) or near your lungs or heart (which can affect blood supply to the back).

How it's done. Once the mastectomy has been completed, you're turned to rest on your stomach or side. An ellipse of skin, fat, and part or all of the latissimus dorsi muscle is elevated away from the back and tunneled under the skin and across the armpit to the mastectomy site (figure 9.1). The incision is then closed. This is an attached flap procedure; once in place, the opposite end of the muscle remains connected to the thoracodorsal artery in the back. You're then turned to your back, and the flap is placed over the pectoralis muscle in the chest. If an expander or implant

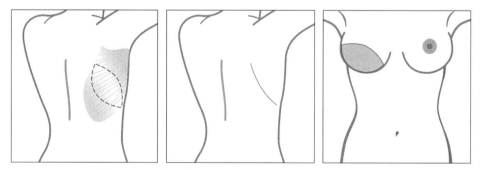

FIGURE 9.1. The latissimus dorsi flap is tunneled under the skin from the back to the chest (*left*), leaving a scar beneath the shoulder blade (*center*). An expander or implant is often added to increase volume (*right*).

TABLE 9.1. Intervals for other flap reconstructions and recovery

Flap type	Surgery and hospital stay	Most routine activities resumed*
Lat flap	4–6 hours; 1–3 days in hospital	4–6 weeks
GAP flap	8–10 hours;† 3–4 days in hospital	4–6 weeks
TUG flap	6–8 hours; 3–4 days in hospital	4–6 weeks

Note: Reflects bilateral reconstruction without complications. Surgical expertise and individual healing affect recovery times.
*Additional time needed to regain full strength and mobility.
†Procedure performed by an experienced two-surgeon team.

is used, the latissimus muscle is sutured onto the lower edge of the pectoralis muscle, creating an instant pocket with overall coverage.

Recovery. Getting back to normal after a lat flap isn't as lengthy, as intense, or as painful as recovery after abdominal procedures, especially an attached TRAM operation. Your upper back may be sore for four or six weeks and will be numb until nerves regenerate. Your underarm will be sore from tunneling the flap around to the chest. You may experience tightness and limited movement and strength in your back for the first few months (table 9.1). A lat procedure doesn't cause significant weakness or interfere with routine activities for most women, but time and the right type of exercise are critical so that other muscles in your back adequately compensate for the loss of the latissimus muscle. Your doctor may recommend physical therapy to help you along. You may experience reduced performance if you cross-country ski, row, rock climb, or engage in other activities that depend heavily on shoulder or back strength.

Potential problems. Back flap reconstruction generally has few complications. If a problem develops, it's more likely to occur in your back than in your new breast. Drains normally stay in place for about two weeks because this flap tends to form seroma, particularly in women who carry excess weight. Necrosis rarely occurs, because the blood supply is very reliable. Bulges sometimes develop under the arm from tunneling the flap to the chest. As the muscle atrophies over time, the bulge shrinks, although it may never disappear completely. Infections are uncommon, but if they occur, they're treated with antibiotics.

Variations on the lat flap. Less common is reconstruction with an *endoscopic latissimus dorsi* flap. This procedure transfers muscle entirely through the mastectomy incision or a small incision under the arm, leaving you with an unscarred back and a shorter and easier recovery. Not many surgeons offer this technique, however. When the back (especially the lower back) has a generous excess of skin and fat, an *extended latissimus dorsi* procedure can be performed to transfer a larger flap to the breast, eliminating the need for an implant but leaving a longer scar. The length of the operation and recovery time are about the same as for a traditional lat flap.

During a *muscle-sparing latissimus dorsi* procedure, an incision is made lower on the back, and the muscle is divided vertically—a small portion is used to create the breast—while the rest remains functional in the back.[2] Patients have good cosmetic results, retain shoulder strength, and experience little or no seroma afterward. Recovery is less painful and requires less downtime than traditional latissimus dorsi reconstruction, and most patients spend just one night in the hospital.

The *thoracodorsal artery perforator* (*TAP* or *TDAP*) *flap* from the back and the *intercostal artery perforator* (*ICAP*) *flap* beside the breast under the arm are muscle-sparing perforator flaps, but neither requires microsurgery because the tissue is moved to the chest under the skin. Because these flaps typically yield only enough tissue for a very small breast, they are most often used to correct post-lumpectomy defects or supplement other reconstruction procedures. A *lateral intercostal artery perforator* (*LICAP*) *flap* also uses skin and fat from the side of the chest near the underarm, usually to improve post-lumpectomy breast defects.

ADVANTAGES OF THE BACK FLAP
- *The standard latissimus dorsi flap procedure is widely available.*
- *It provides a reliable method of reconstruction.*
- *It doesn't restrict or weaken most normal movement after recovery.*
- *Recovery is shorter and less painful than for abdominal flaps.*
- *It reduces the chance of capsular contracture when used with an implant.*

DISADVANTAGES OF THE BACK FLAP
- *It usually requires an implant for a moderately sized breast.*
- *It leaves a lengthy scar down or across the back (unless endoscopic surgery is performed).*
- *The flap skin may be a different hue and texture than the rest of the breast.*
- *May require physical therapy to regain strength and range of motion.*
- *May restrict certain movements.*

I'm the world's biggest chicken when it comes to pain. I asked my doctor what method of reconstruction was the least painful. He recommended using the muscle in my back and a small implant. My recovery wasn't bad, and my new breast is fine.
— Marta

As an aerobics instructor, I didn't want to risk reduced abdominal strength, even though my doctor said I'd be okay after TRAM reconstruction. I read about the back flap in a magazine. I'm glad I did, because my surgery went very well.
— Dee Dee

Flaps from the Buttocks

Posterior, derriere, backside, rump, tush, gluteus maximus. Popular jargon aside, a well-padded bottom can be a prime source for breast reconstruction. The tissue that provides a *gluteal artery perforator (GAP) flap* has a high fat-to-skin ratio and a robust blood supply, producing excellent reconstructive results without needing the muscle. Buttock fat is firm. It forms soft breasts with good volume and projection. You probably have enough gluteal tissue to recreate one or both breasts, even if you're slender and lack sufficient abdominal fat for DIEP or TRAM. You might not be a candidate for this type of reconstruction if you've already had gluteal liposuction.

Except for the donor site location, a *superior gluteal artery perforator (SGAP)* procedure is similar to how a DIEP flap is performed. A slanted elliptical incision is made on the upper buttock, from the outer hip to the intergluteal cleft between the cheeks—the resulting scar is prominent across the top of the buttock, although it falls below the panty line (figure 9.2). A flap of skin and fat is carefully removed where the upper buttock meets the hip—excess fat in the "love handles," the fatty area

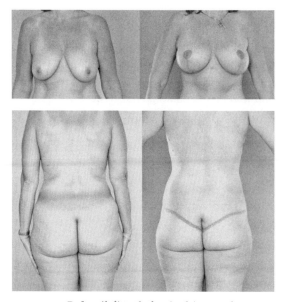

FIGURE 9.2. Before (*left*) and after (*right*) immediate simultaneous bilateral GAP reconstruction, followed by nipple reconstruction and tattoos. Images provided by Dr. Frank J. DellaCroce and The Center for Restorative Breast Surgery, LLC.

just below the waist, or in the lower back can be incorporated into the flap if extra tissue is required—and the gluteal artery feeding the tissue is separated from the muscle. The flap is then reattached to the chest and shaped into a breast. Removing the flap tends to flatten the natural curve of the buttock. This can be somewhat offset by removing the fascia over the muscle, allowing the muscle to protrude into the space created by the flap and restore some of the natural contour.[3] Otherwise, buttock symmetry can be restored by rounding out the donor site with fat liposuctioned from your hips or thighs or by lifting the opposite buttock after unilateral reconstruction.

The less common *inferior gluteal artery perforator* (*IGAP*) procedure removes a flap from the lower part of the buttock through an incision in the crease (figure 9.3). The surgeon must take care to protect the sciatic nerve while dissecting the blood vessels; nicking it can cause irreparable sciatic damage. This is less likely in the hands of experienced IGAP surgeons. The in-the-crease flap uses excess fat low on the buttock to create new breasts. Breast reconstruction with an IGAP flap produces a firmer buttock that results from pulling the skin together when the incision is closed. The surgery scar is hidden in the natural crease beneath the bottom. Few surgeons perform this procedure, preferring to use other flap methods instead.

How it's done. GAP flap surgery is a lengthy and meticulous operation, requiring 8 to 10 hours under anesthesia, even when two surgeons work as a team. You must be turned twice during the procedure. When it's performed as an immediate reconstruction, you are first positioned on your back. Once the mastectomy is completed, you're gently turned onto your stomach so the surgeon can harvest fat and skin from your backside. You're then returned to your back to complete the reconstruction. Delayed GAP flap reconstruction is similar yet shorter, because the mastectomy has already been done.

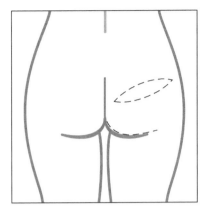

FIGURE 9.3. SGAP reconstruction uses a diagonal elliptical flap from the upper buttock. IGAP reconstruction uses a flap that follows the natural crease beneath the buttock.

Teasing the artery from the muscle can be especially challenging, and in some cases, the superior gluteal artery may be mismatched to the size of the artery in the chest. Few surgeons perform gluteal perforator flaps, and even fewer perform both sides simultaneously. Most GAP surgeons limit this operation to one breast at a time, requiring two separate operations a few months apart to accomplish bilateral reconstruction—that means two surgeries, two bouts with the effects of anesthesia, two recoveries, and a very long overall reconstruction timeline (see table 9.1). If you're interested in bilateral GAP reconstruction, you might want to consider experienced GAP flap surgeons who reconstruct both breasts in a single operation (consult the list at www.breastrecon.com). One surgeon harvests a flap and rebuilds a breast on one side, while the second surgeon does the same thing on the opposite side.

When my implants failed, my only other option was a gluteal flap; I didn't have enough fat in my stomach. Though I didn't look forward to another surgery and recovery, I was pleasantly surprised after my GAP. I was tired for several days, but I had far less discomfort than I did when I had tissue expanders.   *—Kat*

The best thing about the gluteal scar is that I don't have to see it every time I look in the mirror.   *—Sondra*

Recovery. Recuperating from GAP reconstruction is generally less painful and quicker than recovery from TRAM or DIEP reconstruction.

You'll feel a dull ache in the area around the gluteal incisions; that shouldn't keep you from being out of bed for a short walk the day after your GAP surgery. Surgical drains at the chest usually remain for about a week; donor site drains may be required for two or three weeks. Wearing a compression bra around the clock for two weeks, and a surgical compression girdle for two to four weeks helps to prevent seroma and reduces post-op pain by supporting the incision. It may be difficult to sit comfortably or lie on your back. You'll discover which positions are more comfortable until healing occurs. Until nerves surrounding the incision regenerate, the area will be numb. You may notice permanent loss of some sensation around the incision (this happens with all major incisions). The back of your thigh may also be numb for quite some time after an IGAP.

ADVANTAGES OF THE GLUTEAL FLAP
- *There is no loss of muscle function.*
- *The failure rate is low when performed by a skilled and experienced microsurgeon.*
- *The donor scar is usually hidden by swimsuits and underwear.*
- *Even thin women usually have enough buttock tissue for reconstruction.*
- *It produces a firmer breast than tissue from other donor sites.*
- *The recovery is less painful than for abdominal flap surgery.*

DISADVANTAGES OF THE GLUTEAL FLAP
- *The operation is lengthy and complex.*
- *Few surgeons perform GAP flap surgery.*
- *Even fewer surgeons offer simultaneous bilateral GAP flap surgery.*
- *Sciatica may develop if the nerve is damaged (IGAP).*
- *A unilateral flap causes buttock asymmetry.*

Flaps from the Hips

The *lumbar artery perforator (LAP) flap* is a variation of the SGAP procedure, using the "love handles" instead of the upper buttock to reconstruct the breasts. Removing tissue in this area slims the hips and lifts the buttock. It leaves a horizontal scar where the waist meets the upper buttock that is usually hidden by most bathing suits or underwear. LAP reconstruction preserves muscle, so recovery is shortened and less uncomfortable compared to procedures that sacrifice muscle. Hip flaps can be stacked with flaps from other areas to create the desired breast volume (see figure 9.4).

Flaps from the Thighs

The abdomen and buttocks aren't the only sources for tissue flap reconstruction. Thighs and hips can also yield enough fatty tissue to rebuild breasts after mastectomy.

If you carry more weight in your thighs than in your abdomen, a *transverse upper gracilis* (*TUG*) *flap* may be a good option. It's a second-

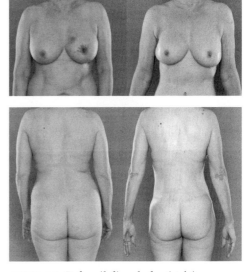

FIGURE 9.4. Before (*left*) and after (*right*) immediate bilateral reconstruction with combined DIEP and hip flaps. Images provided by Dr. Frank J. DellaCroce and The Center for Restorative Breast Surgery, LLC.

ary reconstructive choice when the abdomen isn't an available donor site. Thigh tissue is soft and pliable with a reliable blood supply. Losing part of the gracilis muscle, which works with other muscles to move the leg inward, doesn't affect form or function or cause hernia, as abdominal surgeries can. Because the gracilis muscle is small, it provides only enough tissue for a small to moderately sized breast, less than a flap from the abdomen or the buttocks. Additional volume can be accessed with an *extended* TUG flap from farther back on the thigh or a *vertical upper gracilis* (*VUG*) flap that leaves a more noticeable incision running down the inner thigh. A fleur-de-lis incision combining vertical and in-the-crease incisions may also be used. TUG surgery is less complex than DIEP or GAP procedures, and you don't need to be turned during the surgery.

How it's done. An incision is made just under the groin crease, from the front of the leg to about midpoint under the buttock, through which a crescent of fat and a segment of muscle is removed. The TUG flap is a free flap. It removes part of the muscle surrounding the blood vessels,

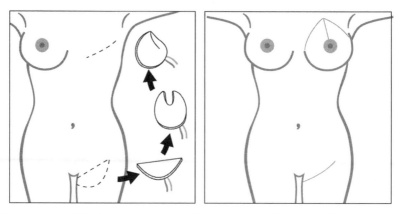

FIGURE 9.5. The TUG flap uses tissue from the inner thigh. The flap is folded over (*left*) and moved to the chest (*right*).

which are then microsurgically reattached to vessels in the chest. The incision is generally well hidden just below the groin crease, and most women don't have a noticeable indentation where the flap was removed. It also has a unique advantage over other flap types: bringing the ends of the crescent-shaped flap together creates an almost perfectly anatomic breast shape with excellent projection. The point of the flap facilitates immediate nipple reconstruction during the initial procedure (figure 9.5). Just a few sutures are placed around the tip of the flap to define the nipple and enhance projection, although some surgeons prefer to create the nipple three or four months later during revision surgery. Because thigh skin tends to be slightly darker than breast skin, later tattooing of the nipple and areola is often unnecessary unless you want additional color. Some women have anatomy that allows a *transverse upper thigh* (*TUT*) *flap*—a true perforator procedure that spares the muscle.

Reconstruction with thigh flaps gives you new breasts and thinner thighs. Performing liposuction of the outer thighs during revision surgery often results in a vastly slimmed down body contour. Unlike abdominal flaps, a TUG procedure is possible even if your thighs have previously been liposuctioned.[4]

Recovery. Compared with recovery from abdominal flap reconstruction, recuperating from TUG flap surgery is quicker and less painful. The location of the incision in the thigh makes for a somewhat awkward recovery because you'll need to refrain from flexing your hip(s) or spreading your leg(s) for the next couple of weeks to avoid putting tension on the thigh incision. Too much thigh movement may delay healing. This shouldn't dramatically affect your final outcome, though it may affect how the incision heals. A compression garment worn on your thigh for several weeks will help reduce swelling. Eventually, *scar revision* may be needed to achieve an acceptable result. You'll be sore for about a week or two, and then you'll begin to improve each day (table 9.1).

ADVANTAGES OF THE TUG FLAP
- *The flap has a reliable blood supply.*
- *The procedure provides an inner thigh lift.*
- *It provides a superior breast shape.*
- *The flap forms an immediate nipple so that nipple reconstruction isn't required.*
- *The incision is well hidden in the groin crease.*
- *The risk of complications is minimal.*
- *There's no noticeable loss of muscle function.*

DISADVANTAGES OF THE TUG FLAP
- *Creates only a small to moderately sized breast.*
- *Initial recovery may be awkward.*
- *The scar may become wider and move lower over time.*
- *The risk for delayed wound healing is increased compared to other flaps.*
- *The risk of lymphedema is increased compared to other flaps.*

Variations on thigh flaps. Tissue can be transferred from any part of the thigh, although not all thigh flaps are cosmetically advantageous at the donor site. The *profunda artery perforator (PAP) flap* uses the fatty part of the upper thigh below the buttock, leaving the patient with an acceptable overall contour and a scar that is well hidden in the buttock crease. The *lateral transverse thigh flap* uses tissue from the upper outer thigh. This free flap operation disfigures the contour of the thigh, leaves a long, obvious scar, and when used for unilateral reconstruction, causes visible asymmetry with the opposite leg.

TUG and PAP flaps are generally considered to be better alternatives. The *anterolateral thigh (ALT) flap* is primarily used to repair injuries or defects in the head, neck, or lower extremities. Although it's easily accessed and has a good blood supply, it's used infrequently to recreate breasts, because taking tissue from the front of the thigh leaves very visible scarring.

CHAPTER TEN

Fixes with Fat

I have one very small new scar on each of my thighs from the entry point. —KELSEY

Surgeons have used *fat grafting* (also called lipofilling, fat transfer, and fat injections) for years to contour sunken facial areas, correct cosmetic hand defects, and plump buttocks and other parts of the body. It's also used by some surgeons as an alternative to implants for breast augmentation (chapter 11). Fat grafting uses excess fat from your belly, thighs, buttocks, "love handles," or behind the knees—anywhere you have it but don't want it—to improve your reconstructed breast. Fat grafting enhances reconstructive possibilities. It's a versatile tool for replacing tissue that was removed during lumpectomy, improving not-so-good reconstruction results, and making a good reconstruction even better (figure 10.1). It's also the primary method of reconstruction after male mastectomy. If your insurance

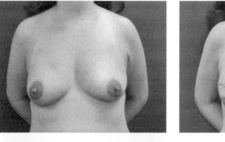
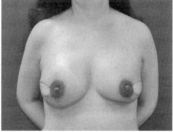
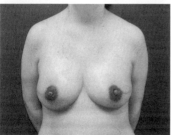

FIGURE 10.1. Before (*left*) and after (*right*) bilateral DIEP flap reconstruction. Subsequent fat grafting (*bottom*) improves overall symmetry, volume, and shape. Images provided by Dr. Minas Chrysopoulo, PRMA Center for Advanced Breast Reconstruction.

covered your mastectomy and reconstruction, it should also pay for fat grafting that improves symmetry or other reconstructive defects.

With earlier fat grafting methods, much of the repositioned fat was *resorbed* (assimilated back into the body). But procedures have vastly improved, making fat grafting more effective and more reliable. Your surgeon transfers fat from a single area—your abdomen or thighs, for example—or from multiple donor sites. (Although fat from the lower abdomen and thigh is sometimes touted as having more stem cells and therefore might be better retained in the breast, multiple studies show that fat retention is pretty much the same regardless of the donor site.) The "from" area becomes slimmer, while the breast takes on soft fullness. The ASPS position on fat grafting is that it is "an effective option in breast reconstruction following mastectomy while demonstrating moderate to significant aesthetic improvement."[1]

Readily available and biocompatible (it's your own living tissue, after all), fat transferred to your new breast can:

- add volume
- smooth contour irregularities and fill in dents
- create or improve cleavage
- further define the inframammary fold
- fill in a sunken area above the breast, especially with implant reconstruction
- hide the edges of implants and camouflage rippling and wrinkling
- soften and improve the texture of previously radiated tissue[2]
- refine the appearance of scars
- improve post-mastectomy pain

Fat grafting may also create a healthy bed of tissue on the chest wall that reduces radiation-induced complications with breast implants. After post-mastectomy radiation therapy, women who had fat grafts injected into the radiated areas of the chest fared well after breast reconstruction with implants. The tissue around the implants healed without problems, the women were free of complications after 15 months, and all of them were quite satisfied with their results.[3]

How It's Done

Removing and transferring fat are relatively simple procedures, but fat grafting involves more than just scooping fat from your hips and plopping it directly onto your breast. Fat grafting is performed after your initial reconstruction, either as a separate procedure or in combination with other revisionary procedures.

The three-step process. Performed as an outpatient procedure under local or general anesthesia, fat grafting involves three distinct stages: (1) harvesting the fat, (2) processing it, and (3) injecting the remaining living fat cells into the breast. (Standard protocols don't exist for any of these stages, and techniques vary widely among surgeons.) Before the fat is harvested, the donor site is infused with a combination of lidocaine (a local anesthetic) and epinephrine (adrenaline) to minimize bleeding. A small puncture, usually a quarter of an inch or less, is made in the skin, ideally in an existing scar, skin fold, top of the belly button, or other inconspicuous spot. A thin cannula (a hollow surgical tube) is then inserted through the puncture, and fat is liposuctioned with a vacuum or retrieved manually; laser or ultrasound liposuction are not the best options for fat grafting, because these methods can damage or destroy fat cells. (Using small cannulas allows reduced points of entry and results in minimal scarring, but somewhat larger cannulas gather more fat—ask your surgeon which will be used for your procedure.) The extracted fat is then either processed in a centrifuge machine or rinsed with sterile saline. Cleansed of cellular debris, blood, and excess fluids that can promote inflammation, the remaining healthy fat is loaded into syringes and injected in minuscule amounts precisely where it is needed in the new breast. Injection points are chosen to be as inconspicuous as possible, often in the inframammary fold or along the edge of the areola.

Unlike tissue flaps that are large areas of fat transferred to the chest with their blood supply intact, fat grafts consist of much smaller particles with no inherent blood supply. Once removed from their blood supply in the donor site, fat grafts must connect to blood vessels in the reconstructed breast to survive. "Layering" the fat into different areas of the breast increases the odds that the grafts will successfully latch onto small blood vessels. It's difficult to predict how much fat will take hold in the breast. A general rule of thumb is that about 50 percent of the fat harvested will be injected, and 50 to 70 percent of that may remain in the breast—the rest will likely be resorbed into the body. So if your surgeon determines that a graft of about 150 to 200 cc is about right, she might liposuction about 600 cc of fat, which should yield about 300 cc to be injected, of which 150 to 210 cc may remain in your breast. Two or more sessions at least three months apart are usually needed for optimal results.

Fatty tissue is fragile and must be handled gently. Unlike cosmetic liposuction, after which removed fat is tossed away, a surgeon's expertise, skill, liposuction technique, and method of introducing the fat into the reconstructed breast affects fat grafting results, and careful handling of fat is an absolute requirement. Your overall health, hormone levels, and the levels of fluid in your fat also influence how much is retained in the breast. Ever-improving procedures are being studied to improve the amount of fat that stays in the breast. Although fat that remains becomes a permanent part of your breast, it continues to function as it would in its original location: increasing or decreasing in volume with your future weight fluctuations.

Recovery. Recovery largely depends on how many donor sites you have and how much fat is harvested. Generally, downtime is short, with minimal discomfort in the breast and mild to moderate soreness at the liposuction area(s) for several days. Most women are up and about the next day and resume work and other normal activities by the second week, when the small stitches that close the liposuction puncture wounds are removed. Recovery takes longer and may be more uncomfortable when more fat and additional donor sites are involved. You'll need to wear a compression garment at the liposuction site(s) for at least two weeks to minimize swelling and accumulation of fluids. You'll also need to avoid compressing your breasts for any reason, including wearing a bra or sleeping on your stomach; you'll be back to wearing regular bras in two weeks when your bruising should resolve. Soreness, particularly at the donor site, may last longer, depending on the amount of fat removed. It may take several weeks before swelling completely subsides. In about three to four months, your breasts will show their final shape and size.

Aside from injected fat that doesn't stay in the breast, complications related to fat grafting are generally few but can involve bleeding, fat embolism, fat necrosis, and infection. Firm lumps that may develop can be anxiety-provoking and should be brought to your surgeon's attention. You may need an MRI or ultrasound to determine whether they are fatty cysts, calcifications, or something else.

Is It Safe?

Fat grafting is increasingly popular for breast augmentation and refining breast reconstruction, but at the time of publication it remains controversial and without consensus regarding the most effective techniques or long-term safety. Some scientists and surgeons worry that hormones, stem cells, and growth factors in the transferred fat could stimulate breast cancer cells and elevate the risk of recurrence and metastasis, particularly in women who are at high risk. Research has produced contradictory results. No controlled, long-term research that follows fat grafting patients for at least 10 years has been done. A mega-analysis of studies on the subject concluded that, "at this point, there is not enough good data to make a definitive claim about the oncologic safety of breast fat grafting in patients. The best studies thus far suggest there is no increased risk of cancer associated with fat grafting, but these are limited by lack of standardization of surgical technique and fat harvest method, inadequate controls, retrospective analysis, and insufficient long-term follow-up."[4] But mounting evidence is positive, including research at MD Anderson Cancer Center that found similar rates of recurrence after six years among women who had post-reconstruction fat grafting and those who did not (table 10.1).[5] Researchers also identified four other notable findings:

- Recurrence in the breast was not influenced by the total amount of fat injected nor the number of fat grafting sessions performed.
- None of the women who had prophylactic mastectomy followed by reconstruction and fat grafting developed primary breast cancer.
- Women who had mastectomy to treat breast cancer required larger fat grafts than those who had prophylactic mastectomy.

TABLE 10.1. Rates of recurrence after fat grafting

Type of recurrence	Percentage with fat grafting	Percentage without fat grafting
Locoregional (in the breast and surrounding area)	1.3%	2.4%
Distant (other parts of the body)	2.4%	3.6%

Note: Mean follow-up times after mastectomy for treatment: 5 years, 44 months for controls; 73 months for cancer-free breasts.

- Among women treated with hormonal therapy, those who had fat grafting experienced a higher risk of recurrence than those who did not (recurrence rates were low in both groups).

Questions for your breast surgeon before fat grafting:

- How many of these procedures have you done to improve breast reconstruction?
- May I see photos of your prior fat grafting results?
- How much fat will you remove, and from where?
- How much fat can I expect to remain in my breast?
- How many fat grafting sessions will I need to obtain the results I want?
- Where will my incisions be? Will I have visible scarring?
- How long will the procedure take?
- How will my donor site look afterward?
- What improvement can I realistically expect?
- What complications might occur and how will you address them?

In my second stage revision, I had fat grafting to help fill in the areas of one breast that was smaller. I am very thin, so the doctor had to be careful. He did a great job; no one but me would know I used to have slightly larger thighs. I have one very small new scar on each of my thighs from the entry point.   —Kelsey

ADVANTAGES OF FAT GRAFTING
- *Uses your own living tissue.*
- *Improves overall shape and fullness of breast.*

- *Slims donor area.*
- *Less invasive than primary reconstructive procedures.*
- *Surgery and recovery are shorter and easier than initial breast reconstruction.*

DISADVANTAGES OF FAT GRAFTING

- *Liposuction and grafting techniques vary among surgeons.*
- *Amount of fat retention depends on a surgeon's experience and technique.*
- *No long-term (10 to 20 years) clinical studies.*
- *Multiple sessions are usually required for best results.*
- *Calcified fat can cause lumps or irregularities in the breast.*

BRAVA+AFT

If you want reconstruction that doesn't involve implants or tissue flaps, you might be interested in BRAVA+AFT (autologous fat transfer), a reconstructive alternative that uses external expansion and fat grafting to gradually "grow" the breast. (The BRAVA procedure is also used for breast augmentation.) Tissue expanders stretch tissues from the inside; the BRAVA device (a special bra with pressurized plastic domes) is an external expander that stretches tissues from the outside. The overall reconstructive procedure takes 9 to 12 months, about the same time as reconstruction with traditional tissue expanders. Initially, a small application of fat is injected into the chest, so you wake from mastectomy (or after the first stage of delayed reconstruction) with a small breast mound in place. You then wear the BRAVA device for 10 to 12 hours a day, three to five weeks—sustained pressure within the domes gradually expands post-mastectomy tissue, enhancing blood vessel and nerve growth in the process. The next step is fat grafting, with liposuctioned fat transferred to the breast in hundreds of microdroplets. Then you go back to wearing the BRAVA device for another two to three months before having another round of fat grafting. The entire cycle—wearing the domes and having fat grafting—is repeated two to four times, two to three months apart, to obtain the desired volume; radiated tissue may require additional sessions. Each subsequent period of expansion increases the amount of fat that can be injected and successfully retained from a single session of fat grafting.

The longer you wear the BRAVA device, the more fat can be transferred at one time, and the sooner you can complete your reconstruction. Three to five days of recovery are typically needed after each fat grafting session.

BRAVA is low tech and time intensive, but it does provide a less invasive reconstruction alternative. You're a candidate for BRAVA if you don't smoke (or stop for several weeks before and after your procedure), you aren't being treated with Herceptin, and you stop using blood-thinning medications, vitamins, and herbal supplements before your procedure. Although the procedure is covered by health insurance as a reconstructive procedure, the cost of the apparatus isn't. The FDA will continue to view BRAVA as an unregulated device until controlled, long-term studies show that it is effective and safe.

ADVANTAGES OF BRAVA

- *Less invasive than breast implant and tissue flap procedures.*
- *Creates minimal scarring (liposuction puncture wounds rather than surgical incisions).*
- *Creates new tissue, new nerves, new blood vessels.*
- *Liposuction removes unwanted fat and slims donor areas.*
- *Involves comparatively short outpatient procedures performed in a surgeon's office with local anesthetic.*
- *The risk of complications is lower than other reconstructive methods.*

DISADVANTAGES OF BRAVA

- *Lengthy start-to-finish timeline.*
- *Requires multiple procedures.*
- *Grafted fat may develop cysts or nodules.*
- *Domes are cumbersome and must be worn for several hours each day.*
- *Domes and associated equipment are not approved by the FDA or covered by health insurance.*

CHAPTER ELEVEN

Altering Your Opposite Breast

At first, I didn't want to have any more operations beyond my initial reconstruction, but my surgeon suggested a breast lift for better symmetry. I'm glad I did that, because both breasts now closely match. —MANDA

When a plastic surgeon recreates both breasts at the same time, he or she can usually ensure they're of similar size, shape, and position with nicely centered nipples. Unilateral reconstruction presents a different problem: how to achieve balance between your reconstructed breast and your natural breast. An optional cosmetic procedure on your natural breast can help you obtain the best possible symmetry. Your reconstructed breast may not be an exact match, but even natural breasts aren't identical. Often, however, reconstructing one breast and altering the other minimizes differences. Performed during revision surgery or as a separate procedure, this opportunity for a breast makeover is something many women may have long considered yet never pursued. (Health insurance companies that cover mastectomy are required by the Women's Health and Cancer Rights Act to pay for modifications to the remaining breast to achieve symmetry, as part of your overall reconstruction.)

After unilateral mastectomy and reconstruction, you have three alternatives for your opposite breast:

- Leave it as it is. If you prefer not to alter your healthy breast, symmetry with your reconstructed breast will depend on the reconstruction method you choose. A flap reconstruction offers a better chance of achieving symmetry, because living tissue can be sculpted and shaped to more closely match your healthy breast than an implant.
- Surgically modify it. Your healthy breast can be reduced, lifted, or enlarged to match your reconstructed breast.

- Remove and reconstruct it. If you have a high risk for contralateral breast cancer, you may want to consider prophylactic removal of your healthy breast. In that case, you'll have bilateral mastectomy and immediate reconstruction.

If you decide to have a little work done on your natural breast, ask to see your surgeon's before-and-after photos of patients who have had unilateral breast reconstruction and the cosmetic procedure you're considering. Notice how closely (or not) their reconstructed and modified breasts match. Ask about the best and worst results you can expect. Discuss your preferences regarding breast size, how you would like your breast to look, how your nipples will be affected, and options for incision placement.

Breast Augmentation

Augmentation mammoplasty to enlarge the breast with an implant or with your own fat is the most common cosmetic procedure in the United States. You'll need a baseline mammogram of that breast before either procedure, and after your operation, you should continue with routine self-exams and mammography (let the technician know that you have implants or fat grafts).

Augmentation with a breast implant. Augmentation surgery with an implant is similar to the pocket procedure used for reconstruction. If your reconstructed breast has an implant under the pectoral muscle, your augmentation will be done in the same way, with the implant placed directly into a sub-muscular pocket; there's no need for tissue expansion. If you had tissue flap reconstruction, your implant might be placed over or under the muscle for your augmentation, depending on your anatomy. A saline or silicone implant will be inserted through an incision made under the breast, along the bottom of the areola, or in the underarm; the underarm procedure makes for more difficult placement of the implant and leaves a scar that will show when you raise your arm, but it doesn't scar the breast (figure 11.1). A *transumbilical breast augmentation* (*TUBA*) incision is a less common option. A saline implant is inserted through an incision made at the top of the belly button, tunneled under the skin to the chest between the breast tissue and muscle, and fully inflated. No incision on the breast means no additional scarring.

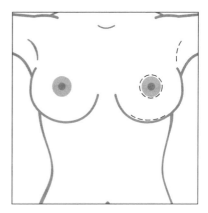

Your chest will feel heavy for several days, and your breast may be bruised, swollen, and sore for two to four weeks. You'll need to wear a support bra or bandage around your chest for at least two weeks to discourage swelling and support the breast until it heals. Be patient if it seems too high or excessively firm; it will drop and soften over the next several weeks as your skin stretches to accommodate the new fullness. Your surgeon may use an elastic bandage above your breast to force it

FIGURE 11.1. Breast augmentation incisions can be made around the bottom of the areola, under the breast, or in the underarm.

down. You may feel tingling, burning, or sharp pains for a few weeks, and your nipple may be quite sensitive; even rubbing against clothing may make it itch or ache—covering it with a round Band-Aid until the sensitivity disappears should help. Within a week most women can shower and return to restricted activities and work that doesn't require lifting, pushing, or pulling, although some women require a few more days of recovery. In three to four weeks you should regain normal range of motion and resume your routine activities.

Aside from the possible risks inherent in surgery and implants, breast augmentation usually causes few problems. A small percentage of women permanently lose some or all feeling in their nipple and areola, and sometimes throughout the breast. If you breast-feed within a year prior to augmentation, you may spontaneously produce a milky discharge for several days after your operation; it's a condition called *galactorrhea* that usually stops on its own. Call your surgeon if your nipple discharges yellow, green, or odd-smelling fluid. These are signs of infection and you may need antibiotics. If you have a silicone implant and you're concerned about breast-feeding in the future and passing silicone to your baby through breast milk, the American Academy of Pediatrics (www.aap.org) says, "It is unlikely that elemental silicon causes difficulty, because silicon is present in higher concentrations in cow's milk and formula than in milk of humans with implants." (Silicon is the natural element upon which silicone is based.)

Augmentation with fat grafting. Many surgeons use fat grafting for augmentation. It doesn't visibly scar the breast and avoids the risk of capsular contracture and other problems associated with implants. You might get a half to a full cup size fuller with a single fat grafting session. Your surgeon may suggest that you pre-expand your breast with a BRAVA device for several weeks before your augmentation to increase the amount of fat that can be grafted or wear the device for a few weeks after the procedure to increase blood supply to the grafts. Augmenting your breast with your own fat is not the best method if you have sagging breasts, poor skin, or you want a significant size increase. Additional fat grafting sessions—opportunities to scale down areas where you think you have too much fat—or an implant would be needed to achieve a greater size increase.

A breast that is augmented with your own fat looks and feels natural but will droop more quickly than an implant. That's because implants lift and support breast tissue, while fat grafts add weight. Using fat allows more versatility. It can be added where it is needed, in the upper pole or inside cleavage, for example, while implants augment only the breast area where they are placed. If you already have an implant in your healthy breast at the time of your reconstruction, fat grafting can improve any rippling, wrinkling, and contour defects you may have. The older implant can also be swapped out for a newer device, with or without fat grafting. Augmentation with fat involves a more lengthy procedure, about three to four hours, than augmentation with an implant.

Although the popularity of no-implant augmentation has skyrocketed, the practice is controversial, primarily because of the concern that fat grafting may hinder screening for breast cancer and that lumps, cysts, and microcalcifications that form in the breast when fat grafts don't survive might interfere with mammography or cause unnecessary biopsies if one of these benign areas appears to be suspicious. The other side of the argument is that calcifications are known to occur in the breast after just about any other breast surgery, including biopsy, reduction, and reconstruction, without worry, and that radiologists know how to read these changes and know when to recommend an additional MRI or ultrasound.

Even though newer, more sophisticated mammography equipment, particularly digital mammography, can better distinguish between benign and cancerous cells, there is always a possibility that you may need a biopsy to determine whether a suspicious area is cancerous. Well-controlled, long-term studies are needed to settle the issue. Meanwhile, a collective analysis of early data on the safety of fat grafting concluded that "surgeons performing breast fat grafting for aesthetic augmentation in young patients with a strong family history of breast cancer must inform their patients of the limited data available on cancer rates in high-risk patients after fat grafting to healthy tissue."[1]

Movement will be more uncomfortable than painful for the first few days after your augmentation procedure. Your breast and donor sites will be swollen and bruised for about three weeks. Most swelling recedes by then, but some swelling can remain for several months. Until your swelling resolves, you'll need to wear a compression garment and surgical bra and avoid excessive lifting, upper body movements, and direct pressure. Most women return to work within a week, although gradually improving soreness may linger for another week. Overall, recovery depends on how much fat is removed and how many donor sites you have. Complications are rare, but bleeding, infection, fat loss, and necrosis are possible.

Breast Reduction

If you're bothered by breathing problems, back pain, or other complications from oversized breasts, *breast reduction* (*reduction mammoplasty*) can make life more comfortable and boost your self-image. Your reduced breast and areola will better match your reconstructed breast and have overall better proportion to your body.

How it's done. Breast reduction is a more complex procedure than augmentation and involves more downtime. It can be done in different ways, depending on your surgeon's preferred technique and how much tissue needs to be removed. You may have a lollipop incision—around the areola and down from the nipple to the bottom of the breast—or an anchor incision, a lollipop with an additional incision along the crease. Alternatively, your surgeon may use a circular incision around the areola: the breast is opened along the incision lines, and excess tissue and skin are removed (figure 11.2). When the amount of tissue to be eliminated is

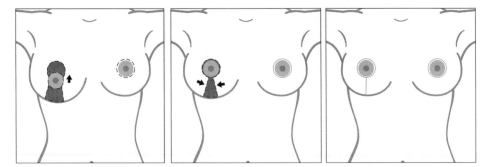

FIGURE 11.2. In breast reduction, excess fat and skin are removed through an anchor incision, and the nipple is repositioned higher on the breast (*left*). The edges of the incision are pulled together (*center*). The newly reduced breast closely matches the reconstructed breast (*right*).

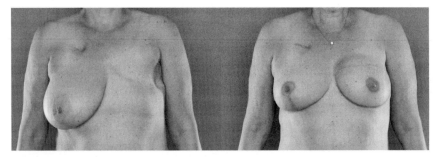

FIGURE 11.3. Before (*left*) and after (*right*) delayed DIEP flap reconstruction and reduction of the opposite breast for symmetry. Images provided by Dr. Frank J. DellaCroce and The Center for Restorative Breast Surgery, LLC.

small, a less invasive incision can be made across the top of the areola or around it, or liposuction may be adequate.

During the operation, the nipple usually remains attached to its nerves and blood vessels on an island of skin that is pulled up and out of the way until the excess breast tissue is removed. If the breasts are large, the nipple may be removed and temporarily grafted to a higher position; this may cause permanent loss of some or all sensation. Once the excess tissue is removed, the nipple is recentered on the breast (figure 11.3). (If your areola is too large for your now smaller breast, it too can be reduced.) The sides of the incision are pulled together, creating a firmer, tighter contour. A surgical drain is placed at the site, and the newly reduced breast is wrapped in an elastic bandage or a surgical compression bra.

Recovery. Breast reduction is a significant procedure and recovery can be uncomfortable, especially in the first three or four days after surgery. After that, you'll be up and around, but restricted from lifting or exerting too much. Bruising and soreness are routine side effects of reduction that dissipate as you heal. Swelling may last up to four months. Bandages are usually removed a few days after the operation, although you'll need to wear a supportive bra around the clock for several weeks. Depending on how you heal and the nature of your job, you may be able to return to non-strenuous work in two to three weeks, but you'll need to refrain from lifting or straining for at least a month. Initially, you can expect to lose some feeling in your nipples and breast skin; feeling returns gradually, but can take three to six months or longer. You may have random shooting pains for several weeks, and numbness in your nipple and breast for several weeks, even up to a year. It may be 6 to 12 months before your breast settles into its new shape. Future weight gains may be reflected in your newly reduced breast.

Potential problems. Disturbing nerves during surgery can reduce sensitivity in your breast. A small percentage of women lose all feeling in their nipples. In very rare cases, the nipple and areola may die from loss of blood. If this occurs, a skin graft is required to rebuild the nipple, which won't have sensation. Your ability to breast-feed is more likely to be preserved when the nipple remains attached to the skin and the milk ducts are left intact. The chance of the ducts being damaged or severed increases if your nipple is removed from your breast during surgery or if you have a lot of tissue removed. Discuss the procedure with your surgeon if you're concerned about the ability to breast-feed in the future. The Breastfeeding After Breast and Nipple Surgeries website (www.bfar.org) provides information and support to mothers who want to breast-feed after reduction surgery.

Breast Lift

All natural breasts head south over time. As gravity takes its toll, tissue loses elasticity, breasts hang lower on the chest, and areolae become larger. A *breast lift* (*mastopexy*) raises and reshapes a breast that sags because of age, excessive weight, pregnancy, hormones, or genetics. If your nipple points downward, a breast lift will reposition it so that it matches the nipple on your reconstructed breast. A breast lift doesn't reduce or enlarge the breast. Small, sagging breasts can be lifted and augmented; overly large breasts can be lifted and reduced.

How it's done. Incision placement depends on the amount of skin to be removed, the position of your nipple and areola, and how much your breast sags. If your breast is small with minimal sagging, a small segment of skin can be removed with an incision across the top of the areola or around it—the scars will be hidden in the border of the areola. A lollipop incision is often used to lift and reshape a moderately sagging breast, while a very large or heavily sagging breast may require an anchor incision (figure 11.4). Once the incisions are made, the breast tissue is tightened and reshaped, and the nipple and areola are appropriately repositioned. Excess skin is removed, and the edges of the incision are sutured together. The same amount of breast tissue is now held together by less skin, so your breast is firmer and sits higher on your chest (figure 11.5). Some or all of your nipple sensation may be temporarily lost, but you can expect it to return as your breast heals.

At first, I didn't want to have any more operations beyond my initial reconstruction, but my surgeon suggested a breast lift for better symmetry. I'm glad I did that, because both breasts now closely match.   —Manda

Recovery. You'll wear a surgical bra for about a week before progressing to an athletic bra without underwire, which you will need to wear

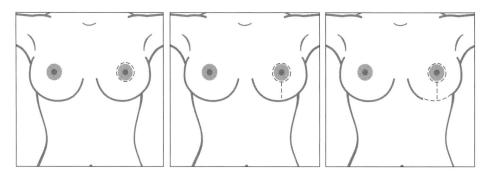

FIGURE 11.4. Breast lift is performed with a periareolar (*left*), lollipop (*center*), or anchor (*right*) incision.

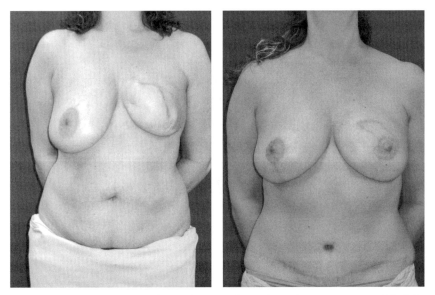

FIGURE 11.5. Before (*left*) and after (*right*) DIEP flap and nipple reconstruction of the left breast after implant removal, and lift of the opposite breast. Images provided by Dr. Minas Chrysopoulo, PRMA Center for Advanced Breast Reconstruction.

around the clock for several weeks. Bruising and swelling will last for up to a month or more. Be very protective of your chest until it heals. Avoid straining, lifting, or exerting pressure on your chest, which can increase swelling, until your surgeon says it's okay to do so. As with other breast surgeries, you should refrain from activities or movements that strain your incisions, and avoid sleeping on your front for at least three to four weeks. Most women can return to work within two weeks and resume full activities in three weeks (table 11.1). Scars from this procedure tend

TABLE 11.1. Intervals for breast modification procedures and recovery

Procedure	Surgery and hospital stay	Back to daily activities
Augmentation		
Implant	1–2 hours; outpatient	1 week
Fat grafts	3–4 hours; outpatient	1 week
Reduction	2–3 hours; outpatient	2–3 weeks
Lift	2–3 hours; outpatient	1 week

Note: May take a while longer before returning to more strenuous activities.

to be very red and lumpy for several months before they fade and become smoother.

Potential problems. Your nipple and breast may be numb for six weeks or more or until the swelling subsides. In some cases, nipple sensation may not return. Until the swelling disappears, your nipples may be off-center or positioned unevenly, and minor revision surgery may be required to improve symmetry. A breast lift shouldn't affect your ability to breast-feed, because the milk ducts generally aren't disturbed.

CHAPTER TWELVE

Final Touches

Creating Your Nipple and Areola

My new nipple is amazing!
—KARLA

You've made it through mastectomy. You have new breast mounds, and unless you kept your own nipples, you're now ready for the final reconstructive step: creating new nipples and areolae. Nipple reconstruction is simple and minimally invasive. It does involve a bit more surgery, but it's minor compared with what you've been through thus far. You're in the reconstructive home stretch.

Icing on the Cake

Nipple reconstruction is a physical and psychological milestone. It completes the restoration of your missing breasts, and for many women, it is the end of the breast cancer experience. Creating a nipple is the icing on the reconstruction cake, although not everyone likes icing. You may consider your new breasts to be incomplete without nipples, or decide to skip nipple surgery because you feel as though you just can't face another procedure or don't consider having nipples to be that important. After mastectomy and reconstruction, some women feel they need a break from surgery, and they wait for a year or longer before having their nipples created.

Perhaps you're concerned about the physical limitations of reconstructed nipples: they'll be permanent bumps on your breast mound that won't react to cold or touch, and they won't change from flat to erect and back to flat again, as natural nipples do, because they'll lack the infrastructure of nerves and small muscles to make that happen. If you have unilateral reconstruction, your new nipple will be standing at attention when your natural nipple isn't. This is something to keep in mind when you're deciding how small or how large you'd like your nipples to be.

Planning your procedure. Nipples can be created during revision surgery while you're under general anesthesia, or anytime thereafter in a separate outpatient procedure under local anesthesia.

Before your plastic surgeon rebuilds your nipples, discuss how you would like them to look: As large as your natural nipples? Bigger? Smaller? Nipples can be made in numerous ways. Ask about your surgeon's preferred method and look at his before-and-after photos. After bilateral reconstruction, your new nipples will be centered at the point of most projection on your breasts. If you're having unilateral reconstruction, decide whether you'd like your new nipple to be precisely centered or slightly off-center to match the nipple on your natural breast. Also consider how much projection you would like to have. At first, your reconstructed nipples will be prominent on your breasts, but eventually they'll flatten. If you prefer protruding nipples, your surgeon can stuff them with fat, an acellular dermal matrix, or a synthetic filler material. If you have microsurgical tissue flap reconstruction, a small piece of your rib cartilage can be used to keep your nipple rigid. During your initial reconstruction procedure, your surgeon removes a bit of cartilage to gain better access to arteries in the chest; it's usually discarded, but it can be banked under your skin, later retrieved and then inserted into your recreated nipples. Discuss this with your surgeon before your flap reconstruction.

Questions for your plastic surgeon:

- How will you create my nipples and areolae?
- How many of these procedures have you done?
- Where will the procedure be performed and how long will it take?
- Will I need an anesthetic?
- Will I have any downtime from the procedure?
- How closely will my new nipple and areola match my healthy breast?
- Where will I have scars, and will they be conspicuous?
- Who will tattoo my nipples and areolae? What is his or her experience?
- What if I'm not satisfied?

My surgeon tried to convince me to "finish the job," but nipples didn't seem important. That was four years ago, and I still don't regret my decision. If I change my mind, I can always have them added. —Karola

Building the Nipple

Most surgeons fashion nipples from a small flap of breast skin. The bow-tie (figure 12.1) and C-V flaps are common, but many other shapes are used, depending on the surgeon's preference.

How it's done. To begin, careful measurements are made to determine the center of the reconstructed breast. The flap pattern for the nipple is then marked on the breast skin. Incisions made along the pattern lines free small flaps of skin and underlying fat. The sides of the nipple flap are folded to meet in the center, and the top part is folded down (figure 12.1). The edges are stitched closed to support the new nipple until it heals. The process takes about 30 minutes for each nipple. Antibiotic ointment is applied to the new nipples, which are then covered with a plastic protector or several layers of gauze with a hole surrounding the nipple. You'll need to wear this protective covering for about two weeks until your stitches are removed. No surgical drains are required. Try not to put any direct pressure on your delicate new nipples for a few weeks until they heal, because that might squash them. Don't shower or involve your nipples in sexual activity until your surgeon gives you the okay. Any mild discomfort (remember, reconstructed nipples have no nerves) can be managed

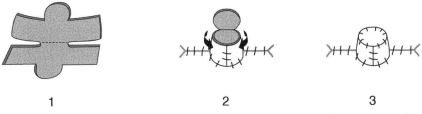

1   2   3

FIGURE 12.1. The most common method of nipple reconstruction involves excising and lifting a flap of breast skin and fat away from the breast. A small portion at the bottom of the flap that remains attached to the breast provides blood supply to the new nipple (1). The side arms are joined in the front and stitched together, forming a platform for the top (2), which is then tucked down and sutured in place (3).

with over-the-counter analgesics. Your nipple needs a healthy blood supply to survive, so avoid smoking, caffeine, aspirin, and other blood-thinning medications (with your doctor's okay) for a few weeks before and after your nipple procedure.

You may be unimpressed with your new nipples when you first see them. They'll be red, swollen, crisscrossed with dark stitches, and covered with scabs after the first week or two. In about a month, soft, natural-looking nipples emerge from the scabby cocoons. It can be a shock when you first see them—they'll be much larger than you expect them to be. Supersizing them is deliberate: they're made up to 50 percent larger than the desired size because they shrink considerably as they heal over three to four months. When the stitches are removed, your new nipple will begin to flatten and shrink so that it is in better proportion to your breast. Once fully healed (in about three months), the nipple and surrounding area can be tattooed to make them darker than your breast skin.

Before mini-flaps were used to rebuild nipples, circular skin grafts from the labia, ear, or inner thigh were commonly used to create the areola. The grafting process creates an additional scar, however, and the donor site remains sore for a week or two. There's a potential cosmetic issue too: if the skin graft has hair follicles, the new nipple may sprout hair. This method isn't necessary for most women (except those with extremely thin breast skin), but some surgeons still prefer to use grafts, so it's worth asking how your nipples will be created before you have the procedure done. If your nipple is made with a skin graft, a protective cover will be sewn onto your breast to shield it for at least a week; during this time you should avoid showering or getting the nipple wet. *Nipple banking*, transplanting the nipples during mastectomy to a blood supply in the groin until they can be transferred to the reconstructed breast, is another option. It is uncommon in the United States, as it is unpredictable and considered somewhat outdated, considering nipple-sparing mastectomy. Another infrequent technique called *nipple sharing* uses a portion of a woman's healthy nipple to create a new nipple after unilateral reconstruction. Even though this provides a perfect color match, it can reduce or eliminate sensation and may affect the ability to breast-feed with the only remaining fully functional nipple. If you're considering nipple sharing, ask your surgeon how your healthy nipple will be affected.

Wow! My new nipple is amazing! It matches my other nipple almost exactly. The only way it could be better is if it had feeling. —Karla

A Colorful Finish

In three months, your new nipples should be healed and ready for cosmetic *tattooing*, the final step in the reconstructive process (figure 12.2). Even though tattooing doesn't create texture or projection, it darkens the nipple and the skin around it to simulate an areola, adding a realistic finish to your reconstructed breast. If you're not ready for tattoos at this point, or you're happy with the way your unpigmented nipples and areolae look, you can simply forgo this optional step or have it done any time in the future.

Tattooing is usually an in-office procedure performed by the surgeon or a member of the office staff. Or consider a consultation with a professional tattoo artist, who is more likely to have a background in art and understand the subtle nuances of blending colors and shading for the most realistic effect. Many provide no-cost services for mastectomy patients. (Some surgeons outsource their nipple tattooing to professional tattoo artists.) Some women take this opportunity to have decorative tattoos instead of more conventional nipple coloring (figure 12.3). Your health insurance may reimburse the cost of having a professional tattoo artist color your areola and nipple, but it's a good idea to check first. If you're going to the trouble of having tattoos, you want them to be as good as possible. No matter who adds the pigment, ask about the individual's specific experience coloring reconstructed nipples, and review before-and-after photos of her work. Speak with some of her previous reconstruction patients, if possible, to see whether they're happy with their results.

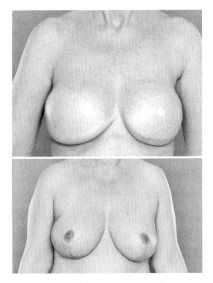

FIGURE 12.2. Before (*top*) and after (*bottom*) nipples are created and tattooed on reconstructed breast mounds. Images provided by Dr. Frank J. DellaCroce and The Center for Restorative Breast Surgery, LLC.

Choosing your colors. Whoever does your tattoos should select the colors with

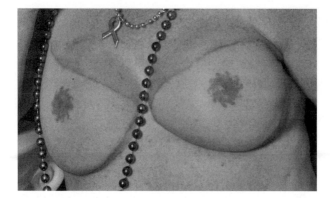

FIGURE 12.3. Some women prefer more artsy tattoos. Image provided by Amy E. Burgess.

your input. Review color samples together to decide which combination would best match your skin tone. After unilateral mastectomy, you can match the color to your natural nipple. If you have bilateral reconstruction, some professionals recommend matching the natural color of your lips. Or bring a pre-op photo of your natural breasts as a reference. Blending two or more shades of beige, brown, tan, or pink sometimes produces the most natural result. Choose a hue that is somewhat darker than your final color—nipple tattoos fade as much as 40 to 50 percent. You might need two or three sessions to apply the full color; layering pigment can help your tattoo last longer.

How it's done. Before your tattoo color is applied, your breast is swabbed with alcohol and the circular outline of your new areola is marked on your breast skin. Check the markings in a mirror before the tint is applied to be sure you approve of the position, shape, and size. If you had unilateral nipple reconstruction, the outlined area should match your opposite areola. If both breasts are to be colored, the markings should be centered. If you don't like what you see, it's easy work to change the markings. If you're dissatisfied with the final tattoo, it's fairly simple to enlarge it or make it darker. It's not as easy to make it smaller or lighter.

Once you've approved the outline, the tattooing can begin. The colors you selected are loaded into an electric tattoo gun that holds sterilized needles. A series of short bursts inject the ink under the skin. The color is a bit shocking when you first see it: it looks like thick, shiny paint. Once under the skin, it will fade to a more subtle shade in a few weeks.

Because of reduced sensation in your breast, you'll probably feel more pressure, tingling, or slight stinging than pain. The longer you wait after your reconstruction, the more likely you'll feel the process, because you'll have regained some sensation. A local anesthesia isn't usually necessary; however, it can be applied if tattooing is too uncomfortable. That's actually good news—it means you've kept or regained feeling in the front of your breast.

It takes about 15 to 20 minutes to color each breast. Your newly tattooed nipples will initially appear brighter, darker, and redder than they'll be when they're healed. (The red is from blood mingling with tattoo color.) You may need to return to fine-tune the color or fill in uneven spots. Your new nipples and areolae will be covered with antibiotic ointment and a light bandage; you should receive instructions for aftercare. There's no downtime from tattooing, so you should be fine to return to work or home or go off to lunch or a meeting. In four or five days, a scab will form over the tattooed area. Take care not to rub, scrub, or pick at it before it falls off on its own, because that can create splotchy, uneven color.

Problems and Solutions

Although nipple reconstructions can fail, serious problems are rare when nipples are made of healthy skin. Complications that do occur usually involve cosmetic issues that are easily corrected. Infections and wound healing problems occur more frequently in radiated skin.

Unsatisfactory pigmentation. Poorly distributed color can create a splotchy, uneven appearance that can be corrected by repeating the tattoo. Nipple tattoos eventually fade; some are only slightly visible after three or four years. While this is a common problem, certain conditions accelerate fading. Nipple tattoos are typically a combination of red and brown, colors that diminish more noticeably than the blues, greens, and blacks used in many body tattoos. The type of pigment and tool used to implant the color can make a difference, and having a local anesthetic can also inhibit color saturation. Your skin quality may also affect the longevity of your tattoo: skin that has been radiated or scarred often doesn't hold color as well. Chlorine can prematurely fade the color, so you'll need to avoid swimming pools and hot tubs for about six weeks after your color is applied. Sun exposure also accelerates fading.

When I first saw my new nipples, I thought my plastic surgeon had made a mistake. They seemed huge in proportion to my breasts. But they kept shrinking as they healed and after a few weeks they were the small nipples I had hoped for. When I later had them tattooed, I thought the tattoo artist had applied too much color. They were several shades darker than I had imagined. Once again, they faded as they healed. Unfortunately, they kept fading, and four years later, they're barely visible. The only thing I can do is have them re-tattooed but I just don't want to bother. —Kim

Poor position. The best way to avoid off-center nipples and areolae is to wait until your reconstructed breast is fully healed before having nipple surgery and to approve the positional markings before pigment is applied.

Nipple collapse. A reconstructed nipple may lose projection and flatten within a few weeks or a few years of surgery. This is more likely when the skin at the donor site is thin, radiated, or scarred. Trauma can also cause a nipple to flatten. The solution is to plump the nipple with an acellular dermal matrix or a cosmetic filler, or repeat the nipple reconstruction process. Stuffing the nipples when they're created avoids this issue, but it also maintains them in the "up" position.

Nipple failure. All or part of a reconstructed nipple may fail if the blood supply is inadequate. The resolution is to remove the necrotic tissue, allow the area to heal, and repeat the nipple reconstruction with a new flap or a skin graft.

Non-surgical Alternatives

If you decide not to have nipple reconstruction, you might prefer adhesive semi-erect nipples, putting them on and taking them off whenever the mood strikes you. Rub-On Nipples (www.breasthealing.com) are one way to have nipples when you want them and forgo them when you don't. If you have one healthy breast and one reconstructed breast, using these products will give you an even appearance. Several companies customize prosthetic nipples in different sizes and skin tones, including the little goose bumps on the areola known as Montgomery's tubercles. Feeling Whole Again (www.feelingwholeagain.com), Reforma (www.myreforma .com), and New Attitude (www.newattitudeprostheses.com) provide customized nipples.

Simulating nipples and areolae with tattoos—adding a smaller dark circle in the center creates the illusion of protrusion. Or look for tattoo professionals who specialize in three-dimensional nipple and areola tattoos. They combine tattoo skills and artistry with subtle highlighting and shading to create a three-dimensional effect, so it looks as though you have nipples even when you don't. In the future, 3-D bioprinting, the same technology that is already creating skin, bone, and heart tissue on demand, may produce living nipples using cells from a patient's own tissue.

PART THREE ○ **PREP, POST-OP, RECOVERY, AND BEYOND**

CHAPTER THIRTEEN

Preparing for Your Surgery

Alone in my house, I cried all day. I was thankful for reconstruction, but I just couldn't come to grips with the reality of losing my breasts. —KATHY

By now, you've done all your research and seen all the photos. You've talked to your surgeon about your reconstruction, and you know what to expect. Your surgery date is circled in red on the kitchen calendar. There's a lot to be done before then, and now's the time to start.

Countdown: Four Weeks to Surgery

Your surgeon will provide a list of pre-op instructions; generally, here's what you can expect within a month of your initial reconstruction surgery.

Finalize payment arrangement. Ideally, you should have your health insurer's payment authorization or have a payment plan in place. If you've petitioned your insurance company for approval well in advance, this should not be an issue.

Consider a recliner. If you don't already have a recliner, consider buying or borrowing one. Finding a comfortable position to rest and sleep can be tricky after surgery. Sleeping in a recliner provides good support, making it easier to sleep in a comfortable position.

Take good care of yourself. Surgery is an assault on the body and its defenses, and fatigue is one of the most common side effects of general anesthesia. Up to this point, you've had to deal with many stressful decisions and issues—all this takes a toll on your mental and physical strength. If you've also undergone chemotherapy, it may have further weakened your resiliency. Now more than ever, your body needs special care to prepare for surgery and improve your ability to recover. This is no time to try a new diet. Eat nutritionally balanced meals with lean protein, healthy fats, and complex carbohydrates. Stay hydrated. Try to sleep for eight hours each night.

Get in shape. Increasing your fitness will help your body weather the stress of surgery. Exercise vigorously for at least 30 minutes a day (45 minutes to an hour is even better).

- Enjoy a brisk walk each morning or evening.
- Walk, swim, dance, try a new exercise video, or engage in other aerobic exercise to boost your immune system and to strengthen your lungs and heart.
- Give yoga a try. Yoga is a particularly effective way to improve the mind-body connection. Regularly stretching the muscles increases flexibility, resilience, and range of motion and is beneficial before and after surgery. Yoga also calms anxiety. It can help to relieve the stress you feel before and after surgery.

Breathe deeply. Our bodies breathe reflexively. We don't have to think about breathing for it to occur. Research shows that deep breathing can profoundly impact well-being and strengthen lung capacity and respiratory function. Consciously inhaling and exhaling expands the lungs, brings more oxygen into the body, clears the mind, and offers new perspective. It's a potent anxiety reliever—an effective way to restore calm after a stressful day or to counter pre-surgery jitters—and you don't need any special equipment. Practice for a few minutes every day. Sit comfortably on a chair or on the floor. Hold your right thumb over your right nostril, closing off the air. Slowly inhale through your left nostril, filling your lungs with air. Hold for five seconds. Release your right nostril, cover the left, and slowly exhale. Now reverse the action: inhale from the right nostril, hold for five seconds, and slowly exhale from the left nostril while covering the right. Repeat this cycle four more times.

Prepare emotionally. Well-documented studies show that people who are emotionally prepared for surgery have less pain and heal sooner. Deal with stress and anxiety proactively. Try deep breathing, meditation, or exercise. Relaxation tapes and positive visualization are also helpful. *Prepare for Surgery, Heal Faster* by Peggy Huddleston is an excellent resource. Or try journaling. Sometimes it's easier to express your feelings to a non-judgmental piece of paper or a computer screen. It's also satisfying. You might be surprised at the depth of perspective it provides.

> *Alone in my house, I cried all day. I was thankful for reconstruction, but I just couldn't come to grips with the reality of losing my breasts. My husband became so frustrated when he couldn't comfort me, he broke down and cried, too. That was the day I decided I was done crying.* —Kathy

Schedule time off from work. Notify your workplace of your upcoming absence and when you think you might return. You don't need to reveal the exact nature of your surgery if you don't feel comfortable doing so, but you should advise your supervisor or boss that you'll be gone and may need to work partial days when you return, particularly if your job is stressful or physically demanding.

Stop smoking. You must be free of nicotine for at least three or four weeks before and after your surgery; if you continue to smoke, your surgery may be delayed. That means no cigarettes, chewing tobacco, nicotine patches, nicotine gum, or other nicotine products. You also need to stay away from secondhand smoke. Ask your primary physician for helpful medication and check out the information at www.smokefree.gov. This could be the push you need to quit for good.

Two Weeks before Surgery

Understand your instructions. Your surgeon (or the nurse) will explain pre-op instructions. Before your surgery, be clear about:

- how long your surgery will last
- how long you'll stay in the hospital
- which medications you should stop taking before surgery, and those you'll need once you return home

You'll receive postoperative instructions when you are discharged from the hospital.

Have pre-op testing. Within a month of your operation, your surgeon will order routine preliminary tests to make sure you're healthy enough for surgery. This might include a blood test to check your red and white blood cell counts, a chest x-ray, and an electrocardiogram to check your heart rhythm. Your surgeon may also request additional tests, including an MRI or a CT scan of your donor site, depending on your overall health, age, and reconstructive procedure.

Recruit help. Never underestimate the power and support of those who care about you. Recruit loved ones to care for your children, pets, and home during your hospital stay and recovery. Let others help. When friends ask how they can help, suggest they babysit your kids, grocery shop, mow the lawn, run other errands, schedule a meal brigade, or drive you to doctor appointments. Schedule a cleaning service, if you need to. Arrange for someone to drive you to the hospital and take you home. Once home, you'll need someone to stay with you for at least the first 48 hours and for several days if you have abdominal surgery.

Discontinue certain medications or supplements. Your surgeon will tell you which, if any, medications, vitamins, herbs, or supplements might interfere with anesthesia or increase bleeding and should be stopped a few weeks before and after your surgery. Taking aspirin, ibuprofen, or naproxen, which can thin the blood and inhibit clotting, is a definite no-no at least two weeks before and after surgery. You'll also need to stay away from medications that contain these ingredients, including many common non-prescription medications such as Advil, Aleve, Alka-Seltzer, Motrin, and others. When in doubt, read the label. Tylenol (acetaminophen) is usually okay for headaches, sore muscles, or other minor to moderate pains. If you're taking Coumadin or another blood thinner, your doctor may request a blood test just before your surgery to make sure your blood clots sufficiently. If you're taking tamoxifen or hormone replacement therapy, your doctor might advise you to temporarily stop before and after your surgery, as both have the potential to promote bleeding and swelling.

Donate blood. Blood loss is minimized during reconstructive surgery and transfusions aren't usually required. If you have a history of bleeding problems, your surgeon will discuss the option to give blood. In the unlikely event that you'll need it, your own blood will be used rather than donor blood.

Go shopping. If you want to wear something more personal than a generic hospital garment, one option is to buy an Annie and Isabel hospital gown (www.annieandisabel.com). Designed by two nurses, the gowns have an inside pocket, snap at the shoulders for easy access to surgery sites, and conform to hospital standards. Some surgeons advise their patients about the type of surgical bra they should buy and bring to the hospital. Most hospitals, however, provide surgical bras; many use the Elizabeth Pink Surgical Bra (www.BFFLco.com), which accommodates surgical drains. If your surgeon prefers a different type of bra, consider ordering a special belt or camisole designed to hold your drains (described in chapter 15). This is also a good time to shop for comfy camisoles, new pajamas, or loose clothing that fastens in the front. If you have abdominal surgery with your reconstruction, some patients suggest buying underwear and sweatpants a size or two larger than you normally wear to accommodate swelling and the compression girdle that you'll need to wear for several weeks.

Fill prescriptions. If you think you'll have trouble getting to sleep the night before your surgery, request a mild sleeping medication. It's a good idea to have prescriptions for post-op pain medication and antibiotics filled now, so that you'll have them when you get home. After your surgery, it will be painful to press down sufficiently to open childproof lids, so ask your pharmacist to use a different type of lid.

One Week to Go

Pamper yourself. Now is a great time to get your hair cut and colored, have a facial, or engage in your favorite self-indulgent behavior. Have lunch with friends. Finish that big project at home or at work. Go shopping. Spend special time with your kids. Have fun. Shave your underarms or legs with an electric razor or consider waxing. Avoid razors that could cause nicks in the skin and encourage infection.

Notify your surgeon of any health problems. Between now and your surgery date, notify your surgeon's office if you get a cold, an infection, a fever, cold sores, or other health problem, no matter how minor it may seem. Your surgery may have to be rescheduled if there is risk of infection—it's always better to be safe than sorry.

Talk to your kids. Many women feel better telling their children about reconstruction instead of keeping it a secret. Children know when something is wrong, even if they don't know what it is, and they want to be reassured that their world will remain unchanged. Kids process information differently. Some ask lots of questions, while others aren't interested, so it's a good idea to tailor your explanations to each child's personality and level of understanding. Your demeanor influences their reaction: if they see you're okay, they'll be okay. Keep it simple for little ones, giving them only the details they need to understand why you'll be gone for a few days, and letting them know that you'll be all right. If they don't already know about your breast cancer and treatment, reassure them you're not ill because of anything they did. Some women prefer to avoid using the word "sick," which may frighten children.

Maintain your child's sense of security. If you're emotional around your children, explain that Mommy is sad or angry or afraid but not because of them. Older children and teens will want to know more. They may feel frightened or threatened if they sense that reconstruction is a taboo topic. Reassure them that you'll be fine and that your reconstruction is a way to help restore your breast after mastectomy. Let them know how they can help during your recovery. Arrange to keep your kids' routines as normal as possible.

My four-year-old had already seen me bald and sick after chemotherapy, so when I told him I was going back to the hospital for a few days to get better, he didn't even blink. —Christine

Our puppy had to have surgery after he swallowed pillow stuffing. When I scheduled my mastectomy, I explained that Mommy's boobs had a type of stuffing that could make me sick, so a nice doctor was going to replace the bad stuffing with good stuffing. I would be in the hospital, as our puppy had, and then I would come home and soon be all better. I gave each of my children a teddy bear I said was filled with "Mommy love" that would never run out. Whenever I couldn't hug them, they could cuddle the bears and it would be like me giving them a big squeeze.   *—Cathy*

Catch up, stock up. A little preparation now will make things easier on you and your family when you come home from the hospital.

- Stock up on groceries, particularly items that someone else can easily prepare. Stash a batch of reheatable meals in the freezer, especially if you don't have someone who can deliver meals or shop and cook for you during your recovery. Have small bags of ice or frozen peas on hand to reduce swelling.
- Buy a thermometer if you don't already have one. It will come in handy if you think you might have a fever.
- Clean your house or have it cleaned before you go into the hospital. You won't be able to sweep or push a vacuum for a few weeks.

Prepare for recovery. Do as much as possible now to prepare for recovery.

- Change the sheets on your bed. You'll appreciate cool, clean sheets during your recovery.
- Make a contact list of telephone numbers or e-mail addresses of friends and family who should be notified after your surgery and updated on your recovery.
- Consider asking friends not to call for a few days after you come home from the hospital; having the phone ring just when you drop off to sleep can be disrupting. (Or turn the phone ringer down or off.) You can always initiate calls when you feel up to it.
- Arrange your nightstand with all the things you'll need at home, including pain medication, TV and DVD remote controls, books or

e-readers, magazines, tissues, lotion, lip emollient, and telephone. Baby wipes are handy for the times when you just won't feel like getting up—although periodically getting up and walking around will be good for you. You'll also want to have water and saltines or graham crackers handy for taking pain medication during the night. Keep a digital tablet, journal and pen, or small tape recorder handy if you're inclined to document your thoughts.

- Reposition bathroom and kitchen counter items so you can get to them without reaching—you'll need to avoid lifting or stretching your arms over your head for a while. If you're having an abdominal flap, reposition items that are under cabinets and on low shelves, so that you can get to them without bending.

The Day before Surgery

Strip your nails. Your fingernails should be *au naturel* when you go into surgery. Polish and acrylic nails can reduce the effectiveness of the fingertip sensor that your anesthesiologist will use to monitor your blood oxygen levels. Toe polish is probably okay, because you'll be wearing socks in the OR, but ask your surgeon to be sure.

Relax in your favorite way. See a movie with friends, have dinner with your family or your favorite person, get a massage, or put on some music and stretch out in a warm bath. Engage in your favorite stress-reducing activity.

Don't shave. Don't shave your underarms or anywhere near an area that is a donor site, because even small nicks can invite infection.

Decide what to wear to and from the hospital. Select a bulky top that doesn't need to be pulled over your head and loose, comfy sweatpants or pajama bottoms, especially if you're having a tissue flap that involves your thighs, abdomen, or buttocks. Wear slippers or flat-heeled shoes.

Pack a small overnight bag. Take moisturizer, lip gloss or lip balm, floss, hairbrush or comb, and any other essentials. The hospital will supply a toothbrush, toothpaste, slippers, and a robe, but you can bring your own if you prefer. It's also nice to pack your favorite music, e-reader, or books-on-tape, particularly if you'll be in the hospital for several days. Remember your health insurance card and personal identification. Some patients appreciate having their own quilt on their hospital bed. Pack a special bag for whomever will stay in the waiting room during your surgery. Include water, snacks, something to read, and a list of family and friends to notify after your surgery.

Stay hydrated. Drink plenty of water and clear liquids throughout the day. Avoid alcohol; it dries the tissues, and you need to be as hydrated as possible for your surgery. It may also interact with anesthesia or postoperative painkillers.

Eat a light dinner. Enjoy a light, low-fiber dinner to discourage post-op intestinal gas and nausea. Surgery is always performed on an empty stomach to avoid the possibility of vomiting. Don't eat or drink anything, including gum, candy, or water, eight hours before your surgery or beyond the cutoff time advised by your surgeon's office. If your reconstruction is scheduled for the afternoon, your anesthesiologist may approve Gatorade, water, apple juice, or other clear beverage. Always follow her instructions.

Make love, if you feel like it. If you're so inclined, there's no medical reason to avoid sex the night before your surgery. It may even help calm your nerves.

Try for eight hours of sleep. With your surgery looming, you'll have a lot on your mind. Try to get a good night's rest. If that's not going to be possible on your own, ask your doctor to prescribe a mild sedative. Don't take an over-the-counter sleep aid unless you have the doctor's okay.

Plant positive thoughts. Before you drift off to sleep, tell yourself that your surgery will be successful, you'll come through it beautifully, and you'll be just fine. Then believe it.

It's Reconstruction Day

Take your regular medication. If your surgeon approved you to do so, take your regular medication with just a sip of water.

Wash your hair. This is the last chance to wash your hair for several days.

Leave it all off. Don't apply wigs, hairpieces, perfume, creams, lotions, or makeup (your natural skin tone is an indication of adequate circulation). Bring eyeglasses (and a case) if you need them; you can't wear contact lenses during surgery, and you won't feel like putting them in and taking them out (or getting up to rinse them) during your time in the hospital.

Leave all valuables at home. Don't take anything you don't need. Leave cash, credit cards, your purse, wallet, watch, and all jewelry, including wedding rings, earrings, and body jewelry, at home.

Talk to someone. Chat with your kids, your spouse, your significant other, or your best friend. It will help to quiet any concerns they're having. It will help you, too.

Leave little notes. If you have kids, tuck a note under their pillow or somewhere they'll be sure to find it, so they'll have a message from you even when you're not there.

Try to relax. It's natural to be nervous before surgery. But you can take steps to calm your thoughts and fears. Plant positive thoughts about your surgery, recovery, and outcome. Take a few moments for deep breathing. Focus on the most positive, beautiful thoughts you can—a happy time, a romantic vacation, or giggling with your children. Visualize a peaceful, happy postoperative you.

CHAPTER FOURTEEN

What to Expect in the Hospital

I began to consider hospitals and doctors as places and people who did things for me rather than to me. —DORENE

Who doesn't get the jitters just walking into a hospital? It's a place we associate with the sick and ailing. Knowing what to expect once you're within those sanitized walls can help calm your fear of the unknown.

Admitting and Pre-op

The hospital will want you to arrive two to three hours before your surgery. Once there, you'll be asked to review and sign a pile of paperwork, including:

- A surgical consent form identifying the procedure to be performed and the name of your surgeon. Be sure you read this and verify the information. Signing the form also means you understand the potential risks of the operation.
- A power of attorney form, identifying your designated appointee to make financial and other decisions on your behalf, if necessary. This can be unnerving, but don't fear. It's a formality for the unlikely event that something untoward happens during surgery.
- Documents concerning your privacy and patient's rights.

A nurse will show you to your room, and you'll change into a hospital gown. She'll weigh you, take your blood pressure, and ask you to remove hearing aids, dentures, prosthetic limbs, contact lenses, or other artificial apparatus.

Each time I enter a hospital, my hands shake and a feeling of dread comes over me. I had to find a more positive perspective to get through my

reconstruction. I began to consider hospitals and doctors as places and people who did things for me rather than to me. I started to consider reconstruction as the process that would put me back on the road to wholeness.
                                                                    —Dorene

While you're waiting, your general surgeon and plastic surgeon will come by for a brief visit before you enter the OR. If the incision lines haven't already been marked on your chest and donor site, your surgeon will draw them now. The anesthesiologist will stop by to discuss your allergies and past experience with anesthesia.

There's always a lot of waiting around before surgery. Free to wander, your mind may go directly to uneasy. Breathe deeply. Concentrate on the positive aspects of your surgery. Mastectomy will remove your cancer (or most of the threat of it), and reconstruction will restore your breasts. If it will make you feel better, discuss your fears with your doctors, your husband or partner, family members, or others who are with you or are just a telephone call away.

I was so nervous the day of my surgery, I broke into a cold sweat. I remember wondering if I would be admitted for heart problems instead of reconstruction, because I was sure I could feel my heart hammering beneath my shirt.
                                                                    —Jasmine

Showtime in the OR

When it's time for your surgery, friends and family will be shown to the waiting room, and you'll be wheeled into the operating room. The first thing you'll notice is the temperature, which is deliberately kept low for the surgical staff. Their tightly woven gowns that protect against bacteria are made with fabric that doesn't breathe, and the room lights generate plenty of heat. Reducing the temperature in the OR also helps to discourage bacteria. A nurse will cover you immediately with heated blankets, and pre-surgery preparations begin. Small sensors will be taped to your arms and legs to monitor your blood pressure and heart rate. The pulse oximeter clipped onto your finger will measure the level of oxygen in your blood.

It's natural to feel anxious at this point, but it won't last long—you'll soon be fast asleep. You'll feel a small sting as the surgical nurse or anesthesiologist inserts a thin needle into a vein on your hand. Through this intravenous (IV) tube, a customized, precise anesthesia cocktail will be administered directly into your bloodstream, based on your weight and the length of your surgery. You'll be asleep before you can count to 10 . . . and maybe before you get to 5.

Modern anesthesia is precise and sophisticated. Yet when patients are asked what they fear most about surgery, many say they're afraid that they'll wake up during the operation. In fact, the anesthesiologist closely monitors and adjusts your sedation throughout your surgery. Monitoring your vital signs and carefully controlling your level of consciousness, he administers a precise dose of sedative to keep you in a deep sleep. Not too much, not too little—just enough.

Once asleep, you'll also receive pain medication, so you won't feel a thing during surgery. A surgical tube in your throat will help you to breathe, and a catheter inserted into your bladder will drain urine. A nurse will wash your chest and donor site with surgical disinfectant. The rest of your body will be draped with sterile sheets, leaving only the surgical areas uncovered. The general surgeon begins your mastectomy as described in chapter 4. The plastic surgeon then moves in to do the reconstruction.

A Peek into Post-op

When your surgery is over, you'll be moved into the recovery room, and your surgeon will let your loved ones know your operation has been completed.

In recovery. You'll slowly wake up as the effects of anesthesia wear off, but you'll be drowsy and will continue to fall in and out of sleep. You'll have an automatic blood pressure cuff, and you may also have an oxygen tube in your nose. If you've had a flap surgery, you might also be hooked to a heart monitor. An IV will drip saline and antibiotics into your bloodstream; the IV remains until you can take in fluids on your own. A nurse will frequently check your vital signs. To ensure your comfort, she'll ask you to assess your level of pain. You'll have a call button or an intercom to summon her whenever you need help.

Compression stockings will help prevent blood clots until you're able to move around—you'll feel a gentle pressure and hear a soft whooshing sound as the pumping machine periodically compresses the stockings to mimic normal circulation. A Doppler probe will be implanted into your new breast so that nurses can closely monitor blood flow to the flap. Your new breasts will be covered with gauze bandages under a surgical bra, and if you had flap surgery, you'll also have a compression garment at your donor site. You may be curious and anxious to see what lies underneath, but unless you get an upside-down peek while a nurse is checking your incisions, you won't see what's under the dressings until they're removed in your doctor's office in a few days.

Initially, medication administered during surgery should handle your pain. If you need it, the nurse can give you additional pain medication and anti-nausea medicine if your stomach is upset. You'll be thirsty, and your throat may be sore from the breathing tube. Ask your nurse for ice chips, water, juice, or throat lozenges. After an implant or expander procedure, you'll soon be moved to your hospital room, usually for an overnight stay. (Some women go home the same day; others remain in the hospital for a second night, depending on how their recovery goes.)

In your room. Anesthesia suppresses the body's ability to function normally. You'll feel weak and tired and your head may feel fuzzy for the next 24 to 48 hours, until its effects wear off. The longer you're under its influence, the harder your body needs to work to recover. Your bed will be angled to elevate your chest, so that you recline in a semi-upright position. If you had reconstruction with an abdominal flap, the lower portion of the bed will be positioned to lessen tension on your donor incision. The urinary catheter will stay in place until you can walk to the bathroom on your own. Constipation is a common problem after general anesthesia; you may not have a bowel movement for three to five days following surgery. Eating lightly the day before your surgery will help to avoid a bloated feeling. Walking, drinking plenty of clear fluids, and eating sufficient fiber will help get you back on track. Ask the nurse for a stool softener if you need it.

Your First Day after Surgery

Now that your surgery is over, it's important to get your lungs back up to full capacity. You'll be given a *spirometer* to help expand your lungs and strengthen your breathing. As you inhale through the mouthpiece, your lungs expand. Exhaling into the device expels the air in your lungs. It's difficult at first, but don't skip this little exercise. Restoring lung strength is an important part of recovery.

Managing pain. Pain is always a concern after surgery, but many women describe their post-reconstructive discomfort as more of a dull, heavy feeling than a sharp or unbearable pain. Of course, a lot depends on the type of reconstruction you've had and your tolerance for pain. To better understand the source of your pain, consider this: You know how annoying a paper cut can be, and that affects only the top layer of skin. Your surgical incision is a paper cut magnified, slicing through skin, fat, and, in some cases, muscle.

Contemporary medicine capably handles post-op pain. Oral medication is usually adequate after implant or expander surgery. Flap surgery is more invasive and requires more substantial pain control, so after that surgery, you'll have a self-medicating pump that regulates the amount of pain medicine you receive—you can use it when you need it, without fear of overdosing. When the pain significantly subsides, you'll be switched to oral painkillers. After tissue flap procedures, many surgeons place a small, round pump that delivers local anesthetic through a thin tube directly to your surgical site. If this adequately controls your discomfort, you won't be as groggy, drowsy, or constipated as you would be with stronger narcotics. The trick to managing pain is to stay ahead of it by keeping a constant, even flow of medication in your system. Allow 15 to 20 minutes for the medication to kick in; dose yourself *before* it becomes unbearable. This is no time to be tough—patients who control their pain heal faster than those who don't. Fresh incisions are tender and sensitive, and applying pressure to them, either internally or externally, will hurt. To your sensitized tissues, a sneeze or cough can feel like a grenade going off. Holding your hand or a pillow gently against your incisions will help. Try to support your incisions in the same way when you get in or out of bed.

Circulation and movement. Movement improves circulation, prevents fluid from settling in your lungs, and helps your system return to normal. As you rest in bed, periodically rotate your ankles and gently stretch your arms and legs. Slowly and carefully flex and stretch as many body parts as you can without causing pain. You'll initially have limited mobility in your arms, and if lymph nodes were removed during your mastectomy, your underarms may be sore. Many movements we take for granted will be difficult and uncomfortable, so be careful and be aware of how you move or stretch your body. Your nurse will show you how to perform gentle exercises for your arms and shoulders, which you should continue to do every day until you've regained full range of motion.

Getting out of bed for the first time will be an effort, particularly if you have an abdominal incision, but the sooner you become mobile the sooner you can go home. It's important to walk around and get your blood circulating, even if just for a few moments. With most types of reconstruction, you'll be encouraged to get out of bed the day after your surgery; after implant or expander surgery, you may be up and walking the same day. Start by sitting up carefully with the help of the nurse. Take a few steps around the room or walk to the bathroom. Try to get out of bed every few hours and take a short stroll or sit up in a chair. It will be difficult and exhausting the first time you get up, but it gets easier as you regain strength. It's also easier to move around when you're not in pain, so for the first few days, be sure you're amply medicated before you get in and out of bed.

The Rest of Your Hospital Stay

Although your health insurance may dictate the length of your stay, all bodily functions must operate normally before you can leave the hospital. Talk with your doctor about staying longer if you don't feel well enough to go home or you develop an infection or other post-op complication.

When it's time to go home, be sure you have the following:

- post-op instructions, including how to care for your incisions
- a list of warning signs for infection or other problems
- directions for managing your surgical drains (chapter 15)

- prescriptions for pain medication and antibiotics (if you don't already have them)
- out-of-hours contact information for your plastic surgeon
- a scheduled follow-up appointment with your surgeon

When you've packed up everything you need and your surgeon has signed your discharge papers, a nurse will help you into a wheelchair and take you outside. (For insurance reasons, patients aren't allowed to walk out of the hospital.) You're on your way home.

CHAPTER FIFTEEN

Back Home

Although I may have felt well during those early weeks, my
body was working very hard in the background . . . healing.

—LIANNE

After surgery, your definition of a good day will change as you recover and regain strength. At first, a good day will simply mean finding a comfortable sleeping position. That will be redefined when you can stay awake, sit up, respond to e-mails or texts, and have dinner with your family. Later, a good day will be when you can lift your arms over your head or go the entire day without pain medication or a nap. One day your cancer, treatment, reconstruction, and doctors' appointments will be behind you. You'll go about your life and forget about your chest, just as you did before your surgery. That will be a good day.

A Timetable for Healing

Just three months after losing his legs in an accident on the track, Indycar world champion Alex Zanardi was up and walking on artificial limbs. Zanardi said of his recovery, "The good thing is that I've turned the first page of that book. Actually, I've finished the first chapter. All of the others are very, very short." Now that's a positive outlook on recovery. If you can view your own reconstruction with the same outlook—the worst is behind you—it will be easier to keep the end result in view.

Once you return home, sleeping or resting will initially take up a large portion of your days. Though you'll be eager to return to your normal routine, don't rush your recovery. Take it one day at a time, and give in to your need to rest. Take advantage of the time to write in your journal, catch up on your reading, watch movies, or nap whenever you feel the need. Listen to your body and be respectful of your need to heal. As your body recuperates, so will your energy and spirit. Don't be frustrated when you can't reach the top shelf or blow-dry your hair. Day by day, you'll get better, and your functionality, strength, and range of motion will improve.

How long will it take to get back to normal? Recovery is such a personal matter, and it's different for everyone. A lot depends on your condition before surgery, the type of reconstruction you have—you'll bounce back faster after implant reconstruction than after a tissue flap—and how much you do to support the healing process. Here's a general description of what you can expect during the first few weeks. Your own recovery may move along faster or take a while longer. And remember to closely follow your surgeon's post-op instructions.

Week 1. Continue performing the arm exercises you learned in the hospital; do them every day to prevent stiffness in your arms and shoulders and to restore range of motion. Take care to move slowly and carefully— no extensive reaching, stretching, pulling, or pressing movements, nothing that puts too much stress on your tender chest tissue; you'll be advised not to lift anything weighing over five pounds—including your children. You'll quickly discover what you can and can't do (table 15.1). You'll feel

TABLE 15.1. Recovery dos and don'ts

10 things you won't be able to do for a while	10 things you'll be able to do
1. Lift more than 5 pounds	1. Take naps
2. Scratch your back	2. Take walks
3. Reach over your head	3. Enjoy TV and movies
4. Sleep on your stomach	4. Work at a computer
5. Exercise aerobically	5. Do range-of-motion exercises (when approved by doctor)
6. Vacuum or sweep	6. Knit, crochet, or embroider
7. Take out the garbage	7. Have meals at home with the family
8. Open childproof or screw-top lids	8. Catch up on your reading
9. Blow-dry or style your hair	9. Use social media to update your status
10. Drive	10. Write thank-you cards

very tired and perhaps lightheaded during your first postoperative week. Even though you may spend much of the day in bed, you can (and should) take short walks down the hall or around the house. If you've had an abdominal flap, your incision will keep you from standing up straight; you'll be hunched over when you walk, until you begin to heal.

It probably won't be your priority for several days, but when you can't wait to have clean hair—it's such a luxury—lean your neck carefully over the sink (if you can do it without pain) and have someone do the honors for you. Your clean hair may need to wait a while longer if you have an abdominal incision and can't manage this. Or ask someone to help you use a dry shampoo that can be brushed away.

It's important to keep your incision(s) clean and dry; a damp dressing encourages infection. You probably won't be able to shower until you return home. If you feel too tired to stand in the shower, try sitting on a shower stool or ask for help. Adjust the showerhead so that the water doesn't beat on your incisions. Wash with a gentle, unscented soap. Be very careful, because you'll still be weak and your incision won't be completely healed. If the surgeon advises you to keep your incisions dry for a while longer, take sponge baths instead, or sit in a half-filled tub if you can do that without immersing any incision. Lightly pat your incisions dry, and leave the surgical tape or surgical glue in place until it falls off on its own or your surgeon removes it. Avoid application of lotions, oils, creams, or powders to your incision, except whatever your physician recommends.

You'll have a post-op appointment with your plastic surgeon within a week of your surgery to check your incisions and change your dressing. (You'll need someone to drive you there and back home.) This is a good time to ask for a copy of your post-mastectomy pathology report.

Know when to call your doctor. It's normal to have discomfort, soreness, and fatigue after surgery. Notify your surgeon, however, if you experience any of the following symptoms:

- chills or a fever
- persistent vomiting or nausea
- pale, blue, or cold fingers, toes, or nails
- increased numbness, tingling, or swelling in your arm or fingers
- redness, swelling, or bleeding from your incision

- increased pain around the incision
- a cloudy discharge or foul odor at the incision
- pain that isn't controlled by your prescribed medication

I always thought napping during the day was such a waste of time. After my surgery, I just gave in to it. I kept a pile of books by the bed. I would wake up, read a little, walk a little, then readjust my pillows and nod off again. How decadent!   —*Mona*

Week 2. Most women find they can do more in the second week, but they're still recovering. After implant surgery, you may be feeling better, and although you may tire easily, you'll probably be able to stay awake longer during the day. Recovery from flap reconstruction will take a while longer. If you've had reconstruction with an abdominal flap, make a concerted effort to stand a little bit straighter each day.

This is the time when it's easy to make the mistake of doing too much too soon. You won't feel like dancing yet, although you should feel better than you did in the first week. Take one day at a time. Move slowly and carefully and give yourself time to gradually get back into the swing of things. Everything you do will take longer and use more energy. You're still recovering—never force your body to do something before it's ready. Add a few more minutes to your daily strolls, until you're walking more each time.

I was tired and fuzzy for a few days after my implant reconstruction; I was okay as long as I took my pain pills. I was so much better by the second week, I decided to shop for groceries. What a mistake! In 10 minutes I was utterly exhausted. I couldn't push the cart one more step. I left it right in the middle of the cereal aisle, got back into my car, and had a good cry.   —*Shelly*

Week 3. By now you should be taking longer walks and staying up most of the day. You may still need a nap or two to feel more alert and less fatigued. Until your incisions heal and your drains are removed, avoid activities that raise your blood pressure, including sexual activity, because excess blood at the incision can cause swelling and hinder healing. If you're well enough and no longer need prescription pain medication, your surgeon may say it's okay to resume driving. Do a test first: sit in a parked car and see whether you're able to open the car door without straining your chest muscles; get in and out, and turn the wheel. If it's too uncomfortable, wait another week before you try again. You'll need to cushion your breasts from the seat belt, whether you're a driver or a passenger. Placing a small pillow or a folded towel between the belt and your chest will do the trick.

If you've had a flap reconstruction, particularly an abdominal flap, you might feel you've hit a recovery plateau about this time. The fatigue, discomfort, and trouble sleeping will catch up with you, and you'll feel weary of it all. After an abdominal tissue flap procedure you may be able to stand straighter by now, even though your abdomen will still feel tight. Continue to take your naps and your walks, do the stretching exercises your doctor recommends, and tomorrow or the next day (or the day after that), you'll notice an improvement.

Week 4. You'll probably be able to resume much of your normal routine by this time (if you haven't already), particularly after implant or expander surgery. If you've had a flap procedure—especially an attached TRAM—or you've suffered healing problems, you'll need extra time to recover and get back to most normal activities. Your abdominal flexibility should continue to improve, but it can take months before the tightness disappears. If you stopped smoking before your surgery, don't resume until your doctor says it's okay to do so. (You've now been off cigarettes for six to eight weeks—a great start to kick the habit!) Be careful the first few times you shave your underarms; they'll be numb if you had axillary lymph node dissection, during which the sensory nerve in the inner arm is often cut. If your new breasts have healed sufficiently, your surgeon may say it's okay to begin wearing ordinary bras.

For the first couple weeks after my reconstruction, I was constantly aware of the tightness in my chest, the feeling that something was different. Then, at three weeks, I felt normal, just like I used to before surgery. It was a big deal; I was getting used to the new me. I felt so good; I made plans to go out on my own, but after just a few hours, I was so tired! I must have overdone it because I needed a nap when I got home; most days I just needed to sit down and relax for a while, and then, I would feel better. I also realized that it was too soon for me to have been driving on my own. Resting after going out seemed to be the routine until almost five weeks to the day, when I started feeling that most of my energy had returned. My mom reminded me that although I may have felt well during those early weeks, my body was working very hard in the background . . . healing. —Lianne

Phantom sensations. As your nerves grow back, you may feel temporary burning, shooting pains, or pins-and-needles tingling similar to when your foot goes to sleep. Some women also experience phantom pains: itching or tingling where the breast used to be. People who lose limbs often report the same phenomenon—it's your brain continuing to process routine signals connected with sensations in the breast. In time, your brain will adjust to the fact that your breast and nerves are no longer there, and the odd feelings will subside and disappear. In the meantime, if your reconstructed breast itches, scratching won't help, because you won't feel it. Try rubbing or scratching nearby, where you do have feeling.

After my mastectomy with DIEP reconstruction, I stayed in the hospital for six days. Pain was minimal; I was off all pain meds, including ibuprofen, within a week. I ate meals with my family from my first day home and slept in my own bed—that was difficult since I had to sleep flat on my back for the first three weeks. My healing was aided significantly by all the help I accepted, including meals, preschool rides, and a cleaning service. I was able to care for myself within 10 days of surgery, and I was completely back to normal within a month. The lifting restriction was the hardest part of the recovery process for me. As a stay-at-home mom, I wasn't able to lift my youngest in and out of the crib. —Jenni

Managing Medication

Take your postoperative antibiotics as directed by your surgeon until you've finished all of them. Manage your pain medication with the following tips:

- Take it when you need it. Studies show that patients who manage their pain heal faster than those who don't. It's more effective to keep a level amount of pain medication in your system than to wait until your pain becomes unmanageable.

- Taper off. When you begin feeling less pain, begin to gradually wean yourself from your pain medicine: take one pill instead of two (or a half instead of a whole). When you think you can tolerate something less, switch to extra strength Tylenol or whatever your doctor recommends.
- Prevent nausea. Take pain pills with milk or food to prevent nausea. If they still make you nauseous, don't take Maalox, Mylanta, Tums, or other antacids, which may negate the effectiveness of the antibiotics. Ask your surgeon for a different prescription instead.
- Be prepared. In the first week or two after surgery, your pain may wake you up during the night. Time your medication so you have one dose just before you go to bed. Keep water and saltines or graham crackers by your bed so you won't have to get up (or wake someone else) to take your medicine.
- Combat constipation. Pain medications and decreased mobility may leave you irregular, and straining from constipation can cause hemorrhoids and adds stress on abdominal incisions. Act preemptively to prevent the problem. Increase your daily fiber intake and stay hydrated. Iron promotes constipation—if you take a multivitamin, use one without iron until your bowels are back to normal. Frequent walking will also help restore your regularity. If your bowels refuse to cooperate, try Colace, Senekot, or other stool softener recommended by your doctor.
- Don't drive until you're no longer taking pain medication.
- Avoid alcohol. It exacerbates drowsiness from pain medication and can sometimes interfere with antibiotics.

Dealing with Drains

Surgical drains are plastic bulbs with long tubing that are sutured under the skin at the incision (figure 15.1). You'll be eager to get rid of these pesky contraptions; however, they aid healing by siphoning off fluids from the surgery sites. Just think what the post-surgical experience was like before someone invented these devices: all that fluid collected by drains would otherwise accumulate in your body, promoting swelling and infection and delaying healing. Until the early 1990s, patients stayed in the hospital until their drains were removed. Today, shorter hospital stays are emphasized and drains are managed at home.

Drains are more annoying than painful, but they can cause soreness where they enter the skin. You'll have one in each breast after mastectomy and if you have a flap procedure, you'll have other drains at your donor site. Your surgeon may remove the drains during your first post-op appointment, but they may need to stay awhile longer, depending on the amount of drainage. You can minimize discomfort and

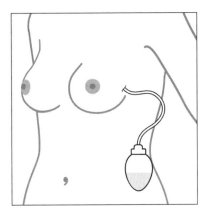

FIGURE 15.1. Fluids from the incision site collect in surgical drains.

awkwardness by immobilizing the drains as much as possible, so they don't pull your skin. Pin the plastic loop on top of each drain to the inside of your robe, shirt, belt loop, or waistband to hold it away from the incision and keep it from swinging or catching on furniture. When you shower, pin the loops to a headband or long shoelace draped around your neck to keep the drains from swinging around. Always position drains below your chest incision so they'll work properly.

Drains are lumpy under clothing. Until they're removed, camouflage with an oversized shirt or sweater is your best fashion strategy. Post-mastectomy garments such as the Softee camisole (www.softeeusa.com) have built-in pockets for drains. When you no longer need the drains, you can remove the pockets and have a soft everyday camisole. Another clever garment (designed by a woman who has been through mastectomy) is the Marsupial (www.turnerhealth.com), a terrycloth belt with attachable drain pouches (figure 15.2).

Emptying the drains. Before you leave the hospital, a nurse will show you how to correctly

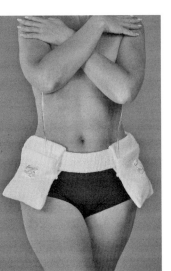

FIGURE 15.2. The Marsupial terrycloth belt comfortably holds drains in pouches. Image provided by Tony Cane-Honeysett.

empty the drains, and provide a measuring cup and a daily log to record the amount of fluid collected. You should measure the contents and empty the drains at least twice a day, 12 hours apart, at the same time each day. (This is a good job for your spouse or partner.) This may need to be done more frequently if the drains tend to fill up. Here's what you'll do:

1. Wash your hands thoroughly with soap and water.
2. Unpin the drain from your clothing or remove it from your camisole pouch.
3. Hold the tubing with one hand where it enters your skin, and slide the fingers of your other hand down the length of it to strip the tubing of all fluids.
4. Open the top of the drain bulb and empty the contents into the measuring container. Be sure to squeeze the bulb to empty it completely. Note the color and characteristics of the fluid. Initially it will be bloody, then yellowish, and finally clear. Notify your doctor if the fluid is cloudy, milky, or foul-smelling.
5. Record the amount of fluid on the log provided by the hospital.
6. Squeeze the empty bulb flat to expel all the air, and close the plug. This creates the suction necessary to remove fluids from the incision. Repin the drain to your clothing or place it back in your pouch.
7. Flush the fluid down the toilet.
8. Repeat the process with each drain.
9. Rinse out the measuring container, and wash your hands again.

Call your surgeon if you have any telltale symptoms of infection in the skin around the drain tube. Once the level of emptied fluid drops below 30 cc (about 2 tablespoons) in a 24-hour period (for each drain), your surgeon will remove the drains by first snipping the suture, then quickly pulling the tubing out of your skin. You won't feel any discomfort if you take a big breath and forcibly exhale as she pulls the tube out.

Those drains were the worst part of my reconstruction. One wouldn't have been so bad, but I had four: one at each breast and two in my hips. One day the tubing caught on a doorknob as I walked by. It yanked sharply against the incision. That hurt!
                                                                    —Kate

*My husband took me to the mall to find a top that would accommodate
the drains. I assured him I would be fine, and then I proceeded to get myself
stuck inside of a blouse while I was alone in the dressing room. I couldn't
lift my arms. All I could do was sit on the chair and alternate between
laughing and crying. At least 20 minutes went by before I was able to find
the perfect amount of yoga, finesse and frustration to free myself from the
shirt. I zipped myself and my drains back into my hoodie and went home
to my pillows.*
                                                                    —Kari

Tips for an Easier Recovery

Much of your recovery depends on your own actions. First and foremost,
be relentless in taking care of yourself. Until you recover, you can't return
to your roles as mom, wife, partner, wage-earner, or caretaker. You have
one priority now, and that is to heal. *You* have to be Number One—not
the job, not the kids, not anyone else. You can't expect to come home from
the hospital and immediately ramp up to normal speed. You needn't treat
yourself like an invalid. Just don't overdo it. Be aware of "patient burnout,"
a malaise that can come out of the blue when you feel sick and tired of
being sick and tired, frustrated that you can't do all the things you want
to, and you just want to be normal again.

Getting in and out of bed. Be very careful when you get in and out of
bed. Those simple, automatic movements we take for granted every day
will be difficult. Think about how you're going to move before you actually do. To get into bed, first sit on the edge and then slowly swing your
legs up. Cover your affected breast with one arm and leverage your position with the other. Move up the bed by scooting your behind from side
to side until you're reclining against the pillows. To get out of bed after
unilateral reconstruction, carefully roll onto your healthy side and use
your unaffected arm to leverage yourself into a sitting position. If you've
had bilateral mastectomy with or without reconstruction, use your legs
and abdominal muscles to first bring yourself into a sitting position, and
then swing your legs over the side. Plant your feet on the floor and slowly
straighten your knees until you're standing. Entry and exit get trickier if
you have an abdominal incision. You'll need someone to help you while

you hold one arm over your chest and the other over your abdomen. If your bedroom is upstairs, consider sleeping on a recliner downstairs until you can easily manage the stairs.

The art of sleeping comfortably. Rest and sleep allow your body to direct its resources toward healing, but finding a comfortable position once you get home can be challenging. If you're used to sleeping on your front or side, it will be several weeks before you're able to do that. You need to sleep in a semi-upright position, as you did in the hospital. This keeps fluids from accumulating in your chest and makes getting out of bed easier. This position may feel a bit strange at first. Many women find it more comfortable to sleep in a recliner that is easily repositioned and easier to get in and out of than a bed.

One way to rest comfortably in bed is to make a nest of pillows. First, position a firm pillow against the headboard or wall—wedge pillows, a body pillow with arm extensions, or a sofa cushion works well—then arrange pillows in front of it to serve as a backrest. Once you're in bed, lean against the pillows behind you. Ask someone to reposition them until you're comfortable. Place pillows under your knees and elevate your surgery-side arm (or both arms if you've had bilateral reconstruction) on additional pillows to take pressure off your chest. Elevate your knees after DIEP or TRAM surgery to relieve tension on your abdomen. If you just can't get to sleep or stay asleep, ask your surgeon for a mild sleeping medication.

Sleeping exclusively on your back and spending so much time in bed can give you a backache. Carefully and gently stretch your back to keep it limber and ward off discomfort. Do isometric exercises in bed, first flexing the muscles along the spine and then releasing them in small concentrated movements. Shrug your shoulders and roll your neck gently from side to side. When you're out of bed, stand straight while you flex your spine, as if you're pushing it against a wall, and then pull it back toward you.

My husband was afraid of rolling into me so he slept in our guest room for six weeks after my reconstruction. It was the only time in our marriage when we slept apart, but it helped. I slept better, and he was close enough to hear me if I needed something during the night.   —*Karina*

Diet and nutrition. It's not unusual to gain weight during recovery. You'll be exercising less and perhaps eating more treats than you normally do, yet now is not the time to diet. Your body will heal faster if you give it the balanced nutrition it needs. Indulge in moderation. Ask friends who provide meals to bring salads or nutritious entrées instead of cakes, cookies, or other high-fat foods. Give your body the protein and nutrients it needs to heal and stay hydrated.

Listen to your body. Don't be afraid to say "not now" if you're not up to a visit or a telephone call. It's good to have time to yourself, to reflect, accept, and just be.

Regain strength, flexibility, and mobility. The therapeutic benefits of exercise have been recognized since ancient times. Exercising moderately for just 30 minutes a day will help prepare you for surgery, and it's absolutely vital for recovery. When contracting scar tissue impairs your range of motion as you heal, restorative movements stimulate circulation and restore flexibility. This is extremely important after mastectomy, with or without reconstruction, and even more so after radiation therapy. Here are some other helpful resources for cancer survivors and post-surgical patients:

The ACS website explains and illustrates post-mastectomy exercises designed to restore range of motion and recondition your chest, arms, and shoulders (www.cancer.org/cancer/breastcancer /moreinformation/exercises-after-breast-surgery).

Your YWCA, local hospital, or breast clinic may offer classes designed for women who have had mastectomy.

If you don't regain full mobility and range of motion in your arm(s) within three or four weeks after your surgery, ask your physician for a referral to a physical therapist or certified exercise specialist who specializes in post-mastectomy physiology and can create a special restorative exercise program for you.

After flap reconstruction, your plastic surgeon will provide a list of additional exercises designed to strengthen and stretch your donor site muscles. Ease carefully into any kind of exercise, avoiding movements that feel too strenuous. It may be helpful to do exercises after a shower, when your muscles are warm and relaxed. The tightness across your chest and in your underarms will improve as you continue your exercise program. Begin cautiously, perform all movements gently and with awareness, and never stretch or pull to the point of pain. You might need to refrain from weight-bearing and more strenuous abdominal exercises for up to eight weeks or more after a TRAM (especially an attached TRAM) or DIEP flap.

Yoga conditions your body before surgery; it's also beneficial once you've recovered sufficiently. Until that time, avoid Downward Facing Dog, handstands, neck postures, and other poses that put pressure on your pectoral muscles. Ditto with stretches that are too intense for the abdomen or other donor site after flap reconstruction. No matter what exercise or movement you do, if it feels weird or wrong, don't do it. Many yoga studios provide specially-designed yoga classes for cancer survivors. Breast cancer survivor and yogi Susan Rosen has an easy-to-follow regimen on her "Yoga and the Gentle Art of Healing: A Journey of Recovery after Breast Cancer" video (www.amazon.com), designed especially for breast surgery patients.

> *Speak to ten different women who have undergone surgeries and you will hear ten distinct stories. Some have wonderful outcomes right away, others struggle for some time; it is plastic surgery after all. Regardless of the outcome or the difficulty, women undergoing surgery and reconstruction will be fine. Our bodies have an amazing ability to heal.*   —Janet

Seeing Your New Breasts for the First Time

It's not unusual to have conflicting feelings about seeing your new breasts. You'll be expectant and hopeful, waiting to see the outcome of several months of planning, surgery, recovery, and waiting. You may feel anxious about what you'll see as you look down at your chest or into a mirror. The reconstruction photos you saw during your research are no longer important, because this is personal. These are your breasts, not someone else's. While most women react positively to reconstruction, some find themselves a bit at odds with their new breasts. Your breasts may be bruised and swollen and not look at all the way you'd hoped they would. Don't be surprised if your surgeon proclaims your breasts to be beautiful. Being far more used to this than you are, she's able to see beyond the swelling and redness to visualize the final outcome. Remember that you're a work in progress. This isn't what you'll look like several months or a year from now, when you're fully healed and your scars have faded. You've suffered a very personal loss. Give yourself time to come to grips with it and grieve for it, if that feels right. The recovery process is temporary. Hang in there and know that the worst is behind you.

When I first saw my reconstructed breasts, I burst into tears. They were horrible! My doctor smiled and said my two little ugly ducklings would grow up to be beautiful swans, and he was right. Nine months later, when I look at my breasts now it is hard to imagine they had such an ugly beginning.
                                                                    —Holly

CHAPTER SIXTEEN

Dealing with Problems

*Compared to my natural-looking right breast, my left
breast was small, hard, and lumpy; they were far from a
matching set.* —JENNI

More women are satisfied with their reconstruction than not, but results
don't always meet expectations and setbacks can occur. Complications
can develop after any surgery, and breast reconstruction is no exception.
Even though serious problems are uncommon, there is always the risk of
infection, a negative reaction to anesthesia, or an unsatisfactory cosmetic
result. When problems linger beyond recovery or become severe, corrective steps can and should be taken. You don't have to live with these issues, and in most cases they can be resolved satisfactorily during revision
surgery or in a minor procedure in your surgeon's office. Chapters 6
through 9 discuss problems specific to expander, implant, or flap reconstruction. Other complications that may occur as a result of mastectomy
or reconstruction are explained in this chapter.

Inherent Surgical Risks

Your risk for postoperative problems is greater after more invasive procedures: mastectomy more so than lumpectomy and mastectomy with breast
reconstruction more so than mastectomy alone. Although most women
experience none of these issues, one or more problems may develop after
your mastectomy or reconstruction.

Bleeding. Excessive bleeding is unlikely, particularly when incisions
are made with electrocautery tools, which use high-voltage electrical current to cut through soft tissue and seal blood vessels. Still, it's important
to heed your surgeon's caution to discontinue using vitamins, herbs, and

medicines that thin the blood. A damaged blood vessel may leak into the surrounding tissue, forming a *hematoma*. Symptoms include pain or a feeling of fullness at the leakage site. The skin may appear dark, as though it's bruised. Your surgeon will want to monitor any hematoma closely, because if it grows too large, it may compress tissues and prevent oxygen from reaching the skin, potentially causing infection, a wound that opens or leaks fluid or blood, or necrosis. A hematoma that isn't resorbed may require surgery to reopen the incision, drain the pooled blood, and reseal the blood vessel. You're at higher risk for a hematoma if you have a bleeding disorder or hypertension. Hematomas can develop if excessive pressure is put on the breast too soon—you fall down, you're elbowed in a crowd, or your partner engages in overzealous squeezing of your new breast.

Seroma. A seroma is similar to a hematoma but involves an accumulation of clear fluid rather than blood. Seromas are less likely with surgical drains and compression garments, but they do still occur. They can be quite small or large enough to cause significant swelling—you may even hear fluid sloshing when you move. These symptoms are sometimes accompanied by pain, skin discoloration, warmth, or redness. Untreated seromas can harden and become infected, requiring antibiotics. If the excess fluid isn't eventually resorbed, your surgeon may need to drain the site with a needle or insert another surgical drain for a few days. If the problem area grows large enough to restrict oxygen supply to the tissue, it may require surgical repair.

Infection. Skin is the body's natural barrier to infection. Anytime the skin is opened, infection has an opportunity to sneak in. Precautionary procedures, such as maintaining a sterile operating environment, keeping your incision sites clean, and dispensing antibiotics through your IV, help protect you during your surgery. Caught early on, most infections respond well to oral antibiotics. Infections that progress may require hospitalization, intravenous antibiotics, and possibly additional surgery to drain off excess fluids. You're more susceptible to infection if you smoke, have diabetes, are obese, are receiving chemotherapy, or have had previous radiation to the chest. Infection is of particular concern when you have tissue expanders or implants, which can become contaminated by bacteria in the bloodstream, and then capsular contracture may develop. For this reason, some plastic surgeons recommend taking preventive antibiotics before any subsequent invasive procedures, including colonoscopy, cosmetic surgery, and even dental work, including teeth cleaning. Treating a lingering infection usually involves removing the implant and *debriding* (removing unhealthy tissue) from the pocket to promote healing, followed by a course of antibiotics. If the implant is removed, a new one can be placed several months later. Contact your surgeon immediately if you develop signs of infection.

My plastic surgeon initially planned to fill the tissue expanders a little after my mastectomy so I wouldn't be completely flat when I woke up. When she attempted to fill them, the breast skin on the right side began to die, so she removed the saline on that side. A week later, I had my first debridement surgery, but the incision popped open again the following week. After another debridement, the incision stayed closed, but my back, stomach, and scar line became red. My entire breast was also red and swollen. I had a cellulitis infection and needed two strong antibiotics for ten days. Then fluid began to leak from my scar, and the surgeon had to remove the expander. Now my left expander is filled to where I want it, and I'm waiting to have a latissimus dorsi flap with implant reconstruction to replace the other expander that was removed.   —Marti

Delayed wound healing. Some individuals take longer to heal than others, particularly when a weakened immune system or chronic health problem leads to *delayed wound healing*. Diabetics, for instance, may heal more slowly from surgery than non-diabetics. Infection slows the healing process, so take every precaution to prevent it. Keep the area around your incisions scrupulously clean and wash your hands frequently.

Your body expends copious amounts of energy during the healing process. You can promote healing by eating a daily variety of nutritious foods. Include sufficient protein, healthy mono- and polyunsaturated fats, and antioxidant-rich foods that supply plenty of vitamins. Be sure to eat enough calories. If you don't have much of an appetite as you recover, eat small nutrition-dense meals throughout the day, rather than two or three larger meals. Hydration is also important. It supports optimal blood circulation that brings nutrients and oxygen to the wound.

Necrosis. Breast skin is fragile after mastectomy. If it's exceptionally thin after the breast tissue is cut away, is handled too roughly, or too many blood vessels that feed the skin are severed, fat in the flap or surrounding an implant may turn dark or harden and die. Your surgeon needs to know about this right away. Depending on the extent of the problem, he may advise a wait-and-see approach or recommend massage for several weeks to soften the area. A small area of necrosis involving the top layer of skin but with healthy skin below (indicating healthy blood supply) may peel away and heal, or it can be surgically removed. If you have tissue expanders, releasing some of the saline may reduce the tension on your skin, giving it "breathing room" to heal. Some surgeons use nitroglycerin paste to improve blood flow or sessions in a hyperbaric oxygen therapy chamber to promote healing by increasing oxygen levels in the tissue.[1] A more serious, although less common, problem is the death of a significant portion of the breast skin or an entire tissue flap. Skin that turns black, indicating that all layers of the skin have died, must be removed. Left in place, it is at risk of developing infection. In this case, an expander or implant would be exposed to infection and need to be removed. (Having a layer of acellular dermal matrix beneath the skin may help to salvage an implant reconstruction.) If an entire tissue flap dies, which is uncommon, a new procedure with an implant or another flap is required to again rebuild the breast when the area heals, which can take several months. Certain risk factors, including having thin skin, a high BMI, smoking, circulatory problems, and previous lumpectomy and radiation increase the risk of necrosis.[2]

My prophylactic mastectomy with nipple-sparing reconstruction went well. My nipples looked good and didn't hurt, but my doctor said some of the tissue was dying—about half of the nipple and areola were necrotic— so I would need to do a few hyperbaric sessions. My nipples healed after half a dozen sessions. They are a different color and look, but I'm okay with that.
—Joanna

*My right DIEP reconstruction was beautiful; my left side was less coopera-
tive due to a compromised blood supply. After a lengthy operation and
another surgery the following day to try to connect the flap artery to a blood
vessel in my underarm, my plastic surgeon said we'd have to wait and see
how my left breast fared. After eight weeks, some of the tissue lived and
some did not. Compared to my natural-looking right breast, my left breast
was small, hard, and lumpy; they were far from a matching set. During an
outpatient surgery, the dead flap tissue was cut away, and I was fitted with
an expander. I am still waiting before exchanging it for an implant. Though
I never thought I'd focus so much attention and time on my boobs, I realize
that in the big picture, fifteen months of surgeries, healing, and waiting is
really not long at all. I waited longer for my youngest to sleep through the
night when he was a baby!*

—Jenni

Lingering Pain

Even though most post-reconstruction discomfort gradually disappears,
some women experience pain or muscle spasms after their incisions have
healed. There's a big difference between ordinary discomfort as healing
progresses and subsequent chronic or intense pain. And though you may
be content to live with cosmetic flaws, you should always seek help for unrelenting pain. Aside from interfering with your physical, emotional, and
psychological well-being, it hinders your immune system's ability to fight
disease and infection. Persistent pain can be caused by scar tissue, hematoma or seroma, chemotherapy, or radiation treatment. Sometimes, lack
of appropriate reconditioning is the cause. A cycle of pain may continue,
for example, when you don't properly rehabilitate your arm and shoulder
after surgery: it hurts, you don't use it, it gets worse.

Women who have axillary lymph node dissection, lumpectomy (especially when tissue in the upper outer quadrant of the breast is removed),
or mastectomy may develop intermittent or persistent chronic pain, most
likely caused by severing or damaging the brachial plexus or intercosto-
brachial nerves that provide sensation to the chest wall, shoulder and upper arm, or sensory nerves in the underarm. This *post-mastectomy pain
syndrome (PMPS)* is rarely discussed as a potential risk of breast surgery.
Loosely defined as pain that remains three months or more after breast

cancer surgery, it isn't well studied, and regrettably, it's not fully understood or acknowledged. Too often, it can be erroneously diagnosed as a routine residual side effect of mastectomy. In many cases, burning, throbbing, or tingling in the arm, shoulder, or chest wall can be mild to moderate or intense, disrupting sleep and quality of life, and restricting the ability to complete normal activities. It may eventually disappear or never go away.

PMPS is more common than you might think. Research shows that 25 to 60 percent of women who have breast cancer surgery develop PMPS, and it occurs more frequently in women under age 40 and in those who have also had breast radiation therapy.[3] If you experience strong or unrelenting pain, you may need a CT scan to determine whether the cause is inflammation, scar tissue, or neuropathy (nerve damage); x-rays and MRI may be used to eliminate other causes. Treatment may include massage; non-steroidal anti-inflammatory drugs (NSAIDs), including aspirin, ibuprofen, and naproxen; or medications that block nerve sensations. A combination of analgesics often proves most effective, and mild antidepressants provide relief for some women. Your doctor can also administer cortisone or a series of anesthetic injections to block sensory nerve paths. Physical therapy and acupuncture can help, as does regular exercise, which prompts your body to release endorphins that block pain signals to the brain. Don't give up and don't tell yourself that you just have to live with the pain. It may take a trial-and-error process to find a solution that works. If pain persists, ask for a referral to a pain specialist, preferably someone who has experience identifying and treating PMPS.

Lymphedema

Women who have lymph nodes removed or have radiation therapy to treat breast cancer have a lifetime risk of *lymphedema*—the risk is higher if you have nodes removed *and* radiation therapy and lower if you have a sentinel node biopsy. Lymphedema is chronic and incurable. When treated early, however, it can be controlled with compression sleeves, special exercises, and therapeutic massage. The National Lymphedema Network (www.lymphnet.org) provides information and support for this condition. There's no way to predict who will or won't develop lymphedema. It may appear soon after lumpectomy or mastectomy or months or even years later. The affected arm may feel heavy, tight, or numb. Lymph nodes that can no longer drain fluid effectively may cause swelling in the arm that may be almost unnoticeable, like fluid retention during your menstrual period. In extreme cases, the arm becomes enlarged from shoulder to fingertips. Contact your doctor at the first sign of swelling, even mild swelling, in your arm or chest after breast surgery.

Be very protective of the affected arm. Keep it scrupulously clean to avoid infection, and protect it from burns, cuts, insect bites, and other injuries. Injections, blood samples, or blood pressure readings should always be taken from your unaffected arm. Historically, women with lymphedema were advised to avoid lifting with the affected arm, but research shows that twice-weekly gentle weight lifting increases strength and decreases symptoms.[4] If you have lymphedema, talk to your doctor before you begin any strength training regimen for your affected arm. Then meet with a fitness professional who is trained in the specific weight-lifting regimen for lymphedema, or ask your local YMCA about the LIVESTRONG program for cancer survivors, which uses the same protocol.

Axillary reverse mapping is a promising surgical approach to lymphedema that uses a blue dye to identify underarm nodes, allowing surgeons to remove nodes that drain the breast and preserve nodes that drain the arm. *Vascularized lymph node transfer* is a microsurgical approach for individuals who don't respond to conventional treatment. It replaces removed lymph nodes with healthy nodes, which then pick up the job of draining lymphatic fluids. Used in Europe and China with some success, vascularized lymph node transfer is gaining interest in the United States, primarily as a companion surgery to DIEP flap breast reconstruction. While the flap incision is open, superficial lymph nodes that aren't the primary source of drainage in the groin or leg are harvested from the donor site and transplanted to the underarm. More surgeons may become trained to offer this surgery—and health care insurers may agree to cover it—if clinical trials show it's safe and effective and doesn't remedy lymphedema at one location only to have it develop at the donor site.

My arm, hand, and fingers began to swell right after my mastectomy. I couldn't bend my wrist or straighten my arm all the way, and it throbbed constantly. It was impossible to hold or carry my baby. I suffered for several months until my doctor sent me to a physical therapist who taught my husband how to do a special massage. We've made this a part of our daily routine. I feel better and my husband is happy he can do something to help. The lymphedema is still there; at least it's manageable now. —Skye

Cosmetic Do-Overs

It would be wonderful if every patient emerged from the operating room with superb results. The reality is that most breast reconstruction requires revision. It's part and parcel of the reconstruction process. Some remedies are easier than others. A minor outpatient procedure may be all that is needed to correct a *dog ear* (puckered skin at the end of a scar) or other minimal cosmetic flaws that mar an otherwise fine breast. Fat grafting can improve many cosmetic irregularities. Lingering complications of larger proportions may require additional revision surgery. If your breast is too big, it can be reduced. If your implant is too small, it can be replaced with one that is larger. A breast can be lifted if it's too low or dropped if it's too high. Displeased with the shape of your belly button after your abdominal flap? Your surgeon can improve this, too. Revision surgery resolves most problems or makes them more acceptable.

While you can't eliminate all possibility of post-recovery complications, taking a few precautions beforehand will help minimize the chance that you'll develop post-op problems and cosmetic flaws.

Choose the most experienced surgeon you can find. Chapter 18 shows you how.

Manage your expectations. Go into surgery with realistic expectations of your outcome, so you won't be surprised when your expanding breast sits too high on your chest or when it doesn't exactly match the opposite side. If you decide to proceed with implant reconstruction even though your surgeon advises against it because of thin or damaged skin after radiation therapy, understand that you have an increased risk of delayed wound healing, necrosis, and other complications.

Give yourself adequate time to heal. Be patient until you're fully healed, because many problems eventually resolve on their own. Reconstructed breasts improve over time. Your flap or implant reconstruction and your scars will look considerably better after a year than they do just two or three months after your initial operation. What is now a misshapen or asymmetrical breast may be fine once the swelling disappears and it drops into its final position.

Decide what's acceptable and what's not. We are our own harshest critics. Subtle flaws in your breast that are all but invisible to your partner may be objectionable to you. (It's interesting to note that many women who are unsatisfied with their reconstructed breasts say their husband or partner thinks they're just fine.) You might decide you can live with the tiny bulge in your new breast or the wide scar on your abdomen, or you might consider them unacceptable. After recovery, perhaps you'll feel that you just can't face yet another procedure, and you're willing to accept what you have as good enough. Or you may want to keep trying to correct flaws that are irksome to you.

Understand what can be changed and accept what cannot. When all is said and done, some problems cannot be fixed. Surgeons can't restore full sensation or eliminate scars, and they may not be able to give you two identical breasts, especially if you've had radiation therapy. Revision surgery may improve the look of your breast, but it might not get it as close to perfect as you'd hoped. At some point, you must accept that your reconstruction is as good as it can be.

Take action. There's no need to suffer in silence. Acknowledging a problem is the first step in treating it. While the thought of additional appointments, procedures, and even minor recovery may be unsettling, discuss your dissatisfaction with your surgeon. He's probably seen and heard it all before, and he can determine whether the problem is likely to run its course or deserves additional attention. If your surgeon approached the initial reconstructive process enthusiastically but isn't keen about handling problems after the fact, look for another opinion if you're unhappy with his response to your concerns.

Address lumps, bumps, and bulges. Although a lump is the last thing a cancer patient wants to find in her new breast, it's not uncommon to find a small lump in a reconstructed breast, particularly after flap reconstruction or a fat graft. Discovering a hard spot can be unnerving, especially if you've already been through the breast cancer experience. Most often, it's a bit of fat that has hardened or died. Some patients develop suture *granulomas*, scar tissue that forms around the internal sutures used to close incisions. Most sutures used for mastectomy and reconstruction dissolve in the body, although your body may have different ideas about that. It will react to any foreign material, even tiny sutures. You may notice a "spitting suture" along your incision; that's a stitch that pokes out through a little bump in the skin. It needs to be removed, because once exposed to the air, it collects bacteria and can cause infection. Your surgeon can easily extract it.

Several months after my TRAM, I developed what I called my third boob—an A-cup-size lump sticking out above my waistline. My doctor said it was the result of tunneling the flap up under the skin. It did finally shrink, but it took almost a year. —*B.J.*

Improving Scars

Scarring is a natural part of the body's healing process and an unavoidable side effect of surgery. Tissue scars when the *epidermis*, or outer layer of skin, is damaged—when you badly burn your finger or get a deep cut, for example. When the *dermis*, the thick tissue beneath the epidermis, is affected—as when a surgical incision is made—the body produces a connective tissue protein called *collagen* to fill in the gaps. It's the body's version of spackle that forms the scar. Scars look different from the rest of your skin because collagen has no sweat glands or pores. When too much collagen is produced, the result is a thicker, more prominent scar.

Why does your friend's mastectomy or donor site scar look so much better than yours? The appearance of a scar is determined by a person's age, genetics, ethnicity, the depth of the wound, and how the incision and underlying tissues are sewn together. If you smoke or have poor circulation, inhibited blood flow at the incision site may make for a more obvious scar. Any scars you have from previous surgeries or wounds are a good indication of how your reconstruction scar will heal.

Mastectomy and reconstruction scars are hard to ignore after surgery, and they never disappear. But most fade to pink after two to three months as collagen and new blood vessels heal the incisions. They become thinner white lines in a year or so and eventually fade into the breast skin; in some women, they're barely visible. Others may remain deeply pigmented, bumpy, or raised. What can you do to minimize scars? Here are a few suggestions to promote healing to make your scars smoother, flatter, and less noticeable.

- Leave the wound alone. To keep the scar line as thin as possible, try not to fuss with your incision or pick at the surgical tape or glue that adhere the edges of the wound together.
- Moisturize. A moist wound heals better than a dry wound. When your incisions close, use a product recommended by your surgeon. Never moisturize a fresh incision, which may invite infection and make the scar worse. Read labels to avoid products that include preservatives, fragrance, or alcohol, which dry the skin. Vitamin E oil may be an adequate moisturizer, but no solid evidence shows that it improves scarring.
- Massage the scar line. As you rub in lotion or cream, massage the scar with your fingertips to stretch and break down fibers beneath the skin. Apply pressure along the length of the scar, then across it. Massage deeply but not to the point of pain. Roll the scar between your fingers each day to keep the tissue soft.
- Give your body adequate vitamin C and zinc. Both aid in wound healing. Taking a good multivitamin that includes both should do the trick, or add several servings of citrus, green leafy vegetables, and foods that are high in protein to your daily diet.
- Protect your scars from ultraviolet light. Scars may darken and become hard if exposed to sunlight or tanning beds during the first year after surgery while your tissue is still healing. Even indirect sun exposure can adversely affect their appearance. Apply a sunblock of SPF 30 or higher, with UVA and UVB protection, and reapply frequently.

- Apply a scar management product. Over-the-counter products won't eliminate scars, but they might help to improve their appearance. You must use them consistently—10 to 18 hours a day for several months—for them to have an effect. You might also consider using a silicone gel or sheet to improve redness and flatten raised areas.
- Re-excise the scar. Surgery won't remove a scar, but it can make it less noticeable.

Some women develop large *hypertrophic scars* that rise above the level of the surrounding skin and remain painful or tender. *Keloids* are thick scars that spread into the skin around the incision. Although anyone can develop keloids, they're more common in dark-skinned individuals. (If other family members develop keloids, you're more likely to have them as well.) Let your surgeon know if you're prone to problem scarring, so he can use a different type of suture, which may help. The International Advisory Panel on Scar Management recommends applying silicone sheeting or gel as soon as an incision is healed to prevent or minimize hypertrophic scars and keloids. The Panel also recommends one or more of the following treatments to improve hypertrophic scars and keloids:[5]

- laser therapy to reduce pigmentation and resurface the scar
- injecting 5-Fluorouracil, a medication for treating skin cancer, into the scar
- injecting corticosteroids to reduce collagen production and temporarily soften the tissue
- dermabrasion, which exfoliates the scar
- injecting fat grafts into the scar
- surgically revising the scar by cutting away the hard tissue and resuturing the incision; this doesn't guarantee that your new scar will be better—hypertrophic and keloidal scars recur about half the time—though it may be worth a try if your scars are bothersome

My scar had a big pucker right in the front of my breast. In about 20 minutes, my surgeon reopened the incision, cut away the scar tissue, and sewed it back up. It felt tight for a few weeks, and then it healed and looked better than before. —Donna

My mastectomy scar is horrible and thick. Even though my doctor revised it, three years later, it's still pretty bad. I knew that was a possibility because I've never scarred well, even from minor cuts. My doctor said it's as good as it's going to get.

—Jean

CHAPTER SEVENTEEN

Life after Reconstruction

My husband kept ignoring my reconstructed breast. I couldn't feel much there, but emotionally, it was important to me to include it in our lovemaking. —ALMA

At last. After months of doctors' appointments, treatment, surgeries, and recovery, your reconstruction journey is over. Your new breasts are in place, and you're ready to move on. You may feel a wonderful sense of closure as you leave your plastic surgeon's office for the last time. Or you might experience sadness or depression, particularly if you've come to regard your surgeon as a trusted friend. This isn't unusual. You've spent a lot of time together during your reconstruction, and now your emotional umbilical cord is about to be severed. Your life is finally getting back to normal.

Adjusting to the New You

It's often said that cancer is a journey. Sometimes we don't realize that until we reach the end of the process and look back. If only hindsight had arrived a little sooner! If you can view reconstruction that way—as an odyssey with an outcome—you'll fare better. When you're uncomfortable, uneasy, or fed up with the reconstruction ordeal, remember it isn't a life sentence. It's a finite experience with a beginning, a middle, and an end. You won't ever forget your mastectomy and reconstruction, but eventually, personal and professional priorities that were shelved during the process will be restored, and your surgeries and recovery will become a distant memory. Your emotional and physical scars will heal, and you'll return to a life without surgeons, weird sleeping positions, or checking your breasts throughout the day. You'll be just fine.

It takes time to get used to the idea of losing a breast. Sometimes it takes a lot of tears, too. Your new breasts will be very different from your natural breasts, and that takes some getting used to, even if they look the same. Most of us can't simply flick an emotional switch and go seamlessly from being patients to non-patients. If you're nagged by depression that you just can't seem to shake, even when your reconstruction is completed, consider the following:

- Put your breast cancer and reconstruction in perspective. It's a bit of a cliché, but cancer does change your perspective. Treatment and reconstruction offer positives for those who are open to them.
- Reprioritize. Actor Michael J. Fox once said, "Illness forces you to get rid of the clutter in your life to make room for the priorities." He was referring to his own fight against Parkinson's disease, but his words ring true for any life-altering experience. Learn—or re-learn—to appreciate life and all it offers. Separate the nickel-and-dime issues, like getting stuck in traffic or burning the toast, from the truly serious. Figure out what's important in your life and move those things to the top of your priority list. Don't feel guilty about items that sink to the bottom and don't get done.
- Don't hide from your feelings. Grief and angst come in all sizes. Some women are emotionally strong, taking mastectomy and reconstruction in stride with a Zen-like approach or an "I don't have time for this" attitude. Others find it impossible to regain any sense of the normal. It's okay—and healthy—to react in the way that's natural for you. At some point, though, you'll get tired of being angry, tired of being sad, and tired of having your life put on hold. The best possible therapy is to acknowledge your feelings and let 'em rip. Then dust off your emotional self and move forward.
- Turn off the negative self-talk. It happens to the best of us: sooner or later those dark thoughts creep into our consciousness. When you catch yourself thinking negatively, replace those thoughts with positive affirmations.
- Create an outlet for your emotions. Deal with your feelings before they begin controlling your life and send you into a downward spiral of adverse emotions. Talk to your partner, a trusted friend or family

member, a member of the clergy, or a local support group. Writing is also therapeutic. Try your hand at poetry or journaling, letting your uncensored thoughts flow freely onto the paper or computer screen.

- Focus on your post-reconstruction life. Appreciate the loss you've suffered from mastectomy but also consider the control you've gained over breast cancer.
- Ask for help. If negative thoughts persist and become more than a temporary funk, consider seeing a mental health professional who can help you resolve troubling issues.

Understand that friends mean well. Your friends will want the best for you, even when it doesn't seem that way. While most people you know will be nothing but supportive, some people have a hard time dealing with illness, surgery, or recovery. Friends may not be able to look you in the eye without crying. You may find yourself comforting them, instead of the other way around. Others may be embarrassed, struggling for the right thing to say. Some might be unable to accept the fact that you're fine, even after your recovery. They'll continue to view you as a victim, even long after you're back to your normal routine. Each time they see you, they'll ask in a soft, sad voice, "How are you?" Don't be surprised if some folks can't seem to draw their eyes away from your chest. Many are curious about mastectomy and reconstruction. When they realize they're talking to your chest, they may become terribly embarrassed. They're all trying to help in their own way. Just take a deep breath and realize they mean no harm.

Remember to laugh. Mastectomy and reconstruction certainly aren't funny, but we can always find humor if we look hard enough. Laughter is powerful medicine. It releases endorphins, sending feel-good messages from the brain throughout the body. Studies suggest that laughter boosts the immune system and reduces pain. One little chuckle or a rollicking belly laugh releases a lot of tension. Ever noticed how quickly kids rebound from sadness? It may have everything to do with laughter—children laugh about 400 times a day; adults, just 25. Find ways to laugh each day. The Cancer Club (www.cancerclub.com) has books, newsletters, and other items that will tickle your funny bone and help you see the lighter side of treatment and reconstruction. Or explore Laughter Yoga (www.laughter yoga.org), a combination of exercises, deep breathing, relaxation techniques, and laughing that help to combat stress and anxiety.

Mend your mind, body, and spirit. You've beaten cancer (or taken steps to prevent it) and completed reconstruction. Now what? Now you experience the sweet relief of returning to your pre-diagnosis life, before the tests and treatments began. Perhaps, like many breast cancer survivors, you feel a new lease on life, one that compels you to find a fresh balance between physical, emotional, and spiritual health. You may feel the need to take better care of your body, not because anything you did caused your breast cancer, but because living with disease gives us such a profound gratitude for the bodies we have. For some, it's cause to reassess or reaffirm beliefs. Perhaps you have a renewed conviction to travel, to change jobs, or to do all those things you've always wanted to do but had to put on the back burner when life got in the way. It's good to look back and reflect. It's even better to look forward and embrace the future.

Your turn to share. If you're inclined to share what you've learned from your breast cancer experience, you can help other women who face the same issues you now have behind you. Whether you spend an occasional hour or get involved full time, you'll find plenty of opportunities to donate your time and insight.

- Let your oncologist and plastic surgeon know that you're happy to speak with other patients who have questions. Many women will welcome your information as they consider their post-mastectomy choices and wonder what reconstruction is like.
- Become a Reach to Recovery volunteer for the American Cancer Society.
- Get involved in annual Breast Reconstruction Awareness Day (visit www.breastreconusa.org to keep up with the various activities).
- Speak to women at your local breast cancer center or support group.
- Donate or raise money for your local breast cancer organization. There are hundreds, if not thousands, of local fundraisers for breast cancer each year across the country. You'll find all kinds of worthwhile

opportunities to raise funds for the cause. Call your local ACS office or search the Internet for "breast cancer charity" to find ways to make a difference.

- If you have an inherited cancer-causing genetic mutation or a strong family history of cancer, consider becoming a volunteer for FORCE.

Back to Work

Returning to work is a giant step on the road back to normal. The workplace can be a positive and caring environment, depending on how close you are to your co-workers and how much they know about why you've been away. Your relationship with your co-workers will dictate how much you do or don't tell them about your treatment and reconstruction. Many women consider their co-workers as extended family. Others prefer not to draw attention to themselves or to be treated differently. If you would rather keep your experience private, when someone asks why you were away, you can simply say it was for health reasons, a family issue, or something similar.

You may need to ease back into the work routine, especially while the pressures and pace of a full day are too taxing. It all depends on the extent of your recovery and the nature of your job: you'll be able to return to an administrative job sooner than to a job as a hospital nurse or daycare center operator. Perhaps you can work flexible hours or part time until you're back up to speed. If your workplace is a source of stress and uneasiness, take time to consider how you'll deal with it before you return. You may need more time to recuperate if you still feel mentally or physically fatigued.

Dating, Intimacy, and Sex

Your medical team gives you information about what to expect before and after surgery, but usually, no one explains about how it might affect your intimate relationship with your spouse or partner. Whether you're single or married, you may worry about how your reconstructed breast will affect your romantic involvements. After months of treatment, surgeries, and recovery, you may feel disconnected from physical pleasure, and intimacy may feel awkward. Lingering effects of cancer treatment can also take a toll on intimacy, long after your stitches dissolve and your incisions heal. It can take time, effort, and patience to resolve these issues and get your love life back on track. Sharing the experience is important to your relationship and will make things easier for both of you.

Lost breast sensation takes some getting used to, particularly if your breasts used to play a starring role in the bedroom. You don't have to give up the pleasure of your breasts, but you may need to redefine how you go about it. Even though your reduced sensation may be disappointing, you can still enjoy your partner's touch if you concentrate on areas that still provide pleasure. Explore the "new girls" together, guiding your partner's fingertips over them and directing attention to the areas where you can feel touch, instead of where you don't.

Although you're the one who goes through reconstruction and recovery, your experience affects your partner as well. You may be perfectly comfortable in your post-mastectomy body and eagerly slip back into the closeness you experienced before your mastectomy and reconstruction. For some women, it's not that easy. Your partner may assume you'll pick up your relationship where you left off, but it isn't always easy to emotionally just snap out of it. Open communication paves the way for the two of you to be more comfortable with your new breasts. Express your feelings and encourage your partner to do the same. It may be difficult to talk about them, but it's important to explain how you feel and what you want. Ask for patience if you need more time to become aroused; explain what feels good and what doesn't, rather than what your partner is doing wrong. Discuss together how you can change your sexual repertoire (if you need to) to satisfy you both. Try not to assume that you're perceived as undesirable if your partner doesn't initiate intimacy; he (or she) may simply be afraid to hurt you or may feel rejected, particularly if you're emotionally distant. Your partner will probably take cues from your own attitude and comfort level with your new breasts. If you're comfortable seeing and touching them, your partner probably will be, too.

My husband kept ignoring my reconstructed breast. I couldn't feel much there, but emotionally, it was important to me to include it in our lovemaking. When I mentioned this to him he said he was afraid he would

hurt me. After we talked about it, we both felt relieved, like a huge barrier
between us had been broken down. —Alma

Take your time. You've been through a lot. You may be eager to get
your love life back to normal, or you may need more time to restore your
sexual health. Allow yourself a period of adjustment to get back in the
groove. Take it slowly if you feel shy, uncomfortable, or apprehensive. Re-
kindle your romantic relationship and let it develop on its own. Spend
time alone together, just being affectionate and doing the things you love
to do. When you don't feel "in the mood," concentrate on enjoying each
other's company. Hold hands as you go for a walk. Start and end each day
with a hug. Make time to share a soothing bath or a romantic dinner. Kiss
and cuddle before you progress to the main event. Work toward being
comfortable with the new you and let nature take its course. Talk to your
doctor if you have vaginal dryness or loss of libido, which can also be affected by chemotherapy and certain medications.

If you feel uneasy or insecure about your femininity when you're un-
dressed, wear lingerie (you'll find a variety of sexy, lacy underwear, even
for mastectomy without reconstruction) or turn off the lights until you
become more comfortable with your new breast. Progress at your own
pace. Remember, the brain is the most powerful sexual organ we have.
You're still very much a woman. Intellectually, you probably know you're
still much more than the sum total of your breasts, but it may take a
while to believe it. If you continue to feel uncomfortable with intimacy,
consider joining a support group or seeking professional guidance; talking with a counselor may be all the help you need to get back to a satisfying
relationship. Let yourself heal, grieve your loss, and deal with the after-
math of your cancer and mastectomy.

When your partner has a problem. If your spouse or partner has been
supportive throughout your mastectomy and reconstruction, you are
truly blessed. Most women find their partners to be a constant source of
reassurance, loving them for who they are instead of what's on their chest.
If the two of you previously shared a strong bond, your relationship is
more likely to weather the stress and emotional upheaval of mastectomy
and reconstruction. If your relationship was already weak, your treatment

and reconstruction can bring you closer together—or drive you farther apart. Some partners are scared silly by the thought of cancer and surgery, but hesitant to discuss their feelings. Others may react with denial, refusing to acknowledge your cancer and reconstruction. Some—hopefully few—may wonder what the big deal is if you're able to have your breast recreated. Early on, ask your partner to accompany you to doctors' visits, participate fully in your reconstruction research, and support you during recovery.

New relationships. Dating presents an interesting dilemma. When and what do you tell your partner-to-be? "Nice to meet you. My left breast came from my belly" or "I'm finally getting my nipples done tomorrow!" may be a bit much when you're introduced. When should you speak up and how much should you say? There is no single right answer to these questions. The best approach is to rely on your instinct to know when the time is right. If you and your date happen to be talking about his mother's struggle with breast cancer, it might be a logical time to share your own experience. In other cases, it may not come up until it becomes very clear that your relationship is heading to the bedroom. Your own comfort with the topic and how you feel about the other person will dictate when you talk about your experience and how much you say. That might be on your first date, when you're getting to know each other, or later in your relationship.

Surveillance after Mastectomy

After mastectomy, it's wise to remain vigilant, but you needn't live your life in fear. Recurrence is unlikely, but leftover cancer cells can form a small lump under the skin, near the mastectomy scar, or in what little breast tissue remains. Some women develop a recurrence in the chest muscle, but that's even more uncommon. A small malignancy in the scar or skin can usually be removed without disturbing the implant or the tissue flap. Excising a larger tumor may require removing the implant or part of the flap. Alert your surgeon immediately if you find a suspicious area or lump in your reconstructed breast, so that the source of the problem, whether it is a calcification, a fragment of dead tissue, or a recurrence, can be identified.

Monitor your reconstructed breast. Breast reconstruction doesn't affect breast cancer recurrence or new tumors, so it doesn't influence whether you should have continuing mammograms. Your mastectomy, however, does. The ACS recommends that "women who have had total, modified radical, or radical mastectomy for breast cancer need no further routine screening mammograms of the affected side (or sides, if both breasts are removed)." This recommendation makes sense, because most of your breast tissue has been removed. (Continued mammograms are recommended after lumpectomy, because you still retain most of your breast tissue.) Some surgeons recommend that women continue to have an annual clinical breast exam, with a baseline mammogram or MRI after reconstruction, especially if you have a genetic mutation that raises your risk of breast cancer, so that any unusual area can be scanned and compared. Continued mammograms are advised if you've had a subcutaneous mastectomy (an early type of nipple-sparing mastectomy that left breast tissue at the base of the nipple and is no longer performed). If you have silicone implant reconstruction, the FDA recommends you have an MRI after three years and every two years thereafter, to detect any rupture.

It's wise to continue examining your breasts each month and to have professional examinations as recommended by your oncologist. If a medical professional has never shown you how to do a breast self-exam correctly, ask your doctor or nurse to demonstrate. Or see the instructive video at the Susan G. Komen Breast Cancer Foundation's website (www .komen.org/bse). Carefully feel along the chest wall, up and over the collarbone, along the mastectomy scar, and in the underarm for any thickened areas or lumps. Look in the mirror for any signs of redness, swelling, or a rash near your scar. Become familiar with the landscape of your new breast. Recognize its irregularities after surgery, so you can distinguish them from any future changes that may occur.

Monitor the opposite breast. If you've had breast cancer in one breast, it's important to continue getting annual mammograms of your healthy breast.

PART FOUR ○ FINDING ANSWERS, MAKING DECISIONS

CHAPTER EIGHTEEN

Searching for Dr. Right

If you can't hug your doctor, you've got the wrong one.

—KAY

You have a primary care physician who oversees your health, a team of medical professionals who coordinate your treatment, and specialists when you need them. When it comes to reconstruction, however, your plastic surgeon takes center stage. You can select your own doctors; that's your right. It's also a responsibility that requires effort on your part. Your choice of plastic surgeons is limited only by the restrictions of your health plan and your willingness to seek out Dr. Right.

Competent surgeons can remove a breast. Rebuilding one isn't as easy. It takes unique skill and experience to tailor reconstruction to each woman's unique needs and doing so in an artful way. Choosing an appropriate procedure is important, but selecting the right plastic surgeon is even more critical to your outcome. A good surgeon is an artist and a sculptor; your post-mastectomy chest is his canvas and clay. Your new breasts are, quite literally, in his hands. He does the work, but you live with it. Some surgeons are good technicians, some are gifted artists. You want one who is both.

Shopping for a Surgeon

Physicians are humans like the rest of us, and being human, they have different personalities, skills, and opinions. You probably wouldn't choose the first financial advisor or realtor you interviewed. It's the same with plastic surgeons. Selecting a doctor is one of the most important personal decisions we make; yet, studies show we spend more time choosing a car. You might randomly find a surgeon from the telephone directory or

Internet and feel relieved to let her make all the decisions about which procedure you should have and what size your breasts should be. That's an easy decision, though it's one you might later regret. If you make the decision to pursue reconstruction, it makes sense to find the most experienced surgeon you can: someone who instills confidence, makes you feel comfortable, and whose work you admire.

It's important to know what a plastic surgeon is capable of giving you. Plastic surgeons usually perform only certain procedures; few are qualified in all methods of reconstruction. When a surgeon downplays one technique or the other, it may be because he feels it's not in your best interest, or because he isn't experienced doing it. Don't expect the best advice about whether you're a candidate for flap reconstruction from a surgeon who only does implant procedures. A surgeon who does implant reconstruction only with tissue expanders may not mention that a direct-to-implant procedure is also an option. Even if you eventually choose the surgeon with whom you first consulted, it's worth the time and effort to make sure he's the one for you. It's a bit like hunting for the right pair of shoes: there's a big selection and not every one will be a good fit. If at first you don't succeed, keep shopping.

> *The mastectomy surgeon recommended a plastic surgeon, and that's who I saw. I never thought of looking for other surgeons. He told me how he would rebuild my breasts and I agreed. Months later, I spoke to another woman who had reconstruction with an entirely different technique that sounded much better. Why didn't my surgeon mention that?*
> —*Lanie*

Five Characteristics of an Ideal Plastic Surgeon

As you consult with different surgeons, look for five important characteristics.

    1. *Skill.* There's no such thing as a typical reconstruction, because each woman is different. It takes skill and experience to rebuild and fine-tune a breast to get the very best result. Assess a plastic surgeon's qualifications, feedback from other patients, photos of her work, and your own confidence in the information she provides.

2. *Compassion.* You're more than a statistic on a chart, and you deserve to be treated respectfully and as an individual. A good surgeon cares about your expectations and willingly repeats or clarifies information, is sympathetic to your concerns, and reacts to your anxiety with compassion. Ideally, you want someone who is proficient with both the technical and the non-technical aspects of care—not one or the other.

3. *Communication.* "My doctor doesn't listen to me" is a frequent complaint in patient satisfaction surveys. Your surgeon should talk with you, not to you, and give you his undivided attention. Choose someone who cares about your concerns and pays attention to what you want, rather than dictating how your reconstruction will be handled. The surgeon should explain terms and procedures so that you can understand them, and should patiently answer your questions even when you ask for something to be repeated.

4. *Rapport.* It's important to find a surgeon you like. You'll have many questions and concerns throughout the process, and you need to feel comfortable voicing them. One surgeon may be too aggressive, another too impersonal for your taste. Your surgeon should never be condescending, abrupt, or rude.

5. *Honesty.* Look for someone who describes what you can realistically expect, rather than what she thinks you want to hear. If you have your heart set on D-cup implants, she should tell you whether your skin can be expanded sufficiently to accommodate that size. Leaning toward a tissue flap? Your surgeon ought to candidly describe what you can expect from the operation and recovery and how you'll look afterward. Think twice if a surgeon promises "You'll be as good as new" or "Your breasts will be perfect." You should be honest, too. Say what's on your mind, rather than what you think she expects.

My surgeon put me at ease by patiently answering all my questions. He smiled a lot, spoke slowly, and explained several different ways the reconstruction might be done. I felt I was talking to a trusted friend. —Cameran

I was so put off by my surgeon, I skipped my last appointment. He seemed more interested in me as his "creation" than as a person with cancer. He refused to accept that I didn't want big breasts. —Alicia

I saw three different surgeons, who recommended three different tech-niques! One wanted to reconstruct my breast with implants, another wanted to use tissue from my back, and the third said I would have better results using my abdominal fat.   —Betty

Your Pre-appointment Footwork

Where do you find Dr. Right? Many hospitals and universities with medi-cal centers have departments devoted specifically to breast cancer surgery, and many have excellent reconstruction staff. Hospital and recovery room nurses are great sources of information and often have firsthand experi-ence with surgeons' work. Personal feedback is always preferable to the "eeney meeney miney moe" selection method. It's always nice to have a report from someone who's already been through reconstruction, prefer-ably involving the same technique you're considering. Ask other women which surgeons they do or don't recommend and why. The FORCE Sur-geon Referral Tool (www.facingourrisk.org) is a patient-based database of surgeons that can be searched by surgeon name, city, state, or type of sur-gery. It puts you in touch with women who are willing to share their ex-periences. Reach to Recovery will also put you in touch with women in your area who'll share their insights into the reconstruction experience and give you feedback about their plastic surgeons (call your local ACS of-fice for information about the program). Or hop online to the American Society of Plastic Surgeons (www.plasticsurgery.org), the largest profes-sional organization of reconstructive surgeons, to search by zip code or name. Check this book's companion website (www.breastrecon.com) for surgeons who offer direct-to-implant or microsurgical reconstruction. Make a list of reconstructive surgeons, and then consult with at least two or three before selecting your Dr. Right.

If possible, choose a physician who specializes in breast reconstruction—some do so exclusively—you don't want your new breasts to be created by a cosmetic surgeon who primarily provides facelifts or other cosmetic procedures and seldom performs breast reconstruction. (Your insurance, particularly if you have an HMO, may require you to use an in-network surgeon.)

Before you schedule an appointment. As a first step, check surgeons' websites or call their offices to ask a few key questions.

- Is the doctor accepting new patients?
- Does the doctor accept your insurance?
- What breast reconstruction procedures does the surgeon perform?
- How much experience does the surgeon have with each procedure?
- Does the plastic surgeon work with a breast surgeon who is experienced with nipple-sparing mastectomy (if that is what you'd like)?
- What is the surgeon's hospital affiliation?

Verify certification. Believe it or not, physicians don't need to be certified to perform plastic surgery. In most states any licensed physician can perform plastic surgery. While board certification doesn't guarantee proficiency, it's the best starting place. To be certified by the ASPS, for example, a surgeon must graduate from an accredited medical school, complete six years of surgical training, including at least three years of plastic surgery residency, successfully complete oral and written exams, and complete continuing medical education. Verify certification for the surgeons you are considering at the American Board of Medical Specialties (www.abms.org).

Schedule a consultation. After weeding out individuals who don't take your insurance, don't provide the procedure you want, or various other reasons, you're ready to arrange consultations with the top three or four surgeons on your list. (Scheduling an appointment early in the day, if that works for you, will give you a better chance of seeing the doctor on time.) Ask the receptionist how much time you'll have in the office—consultation appointments are often scheduled for 30 to 60 minutes—if your consultation will be less than 30 minutes, ask for a longer appointment. The time will fly by as the surgeon examines you and describes various reconstructive procedures. Good plastic surgeons keep busy. If your mastectomy date is quickly approaching, let the receptionist know; she may be able to fit you in. In the meantime, interview other surgeons on your list.

Making the Most of Your Consultation

Your consultation appointment will begin with a review of your cancer diagnosis or treatment, genetic status (if you're pursuing preventive mastectomy), and overall medical history. The discussion should include the reconstructive procedures the surgeon performs and what he thinks would work well for you (and why), based on your reconstructive preferences. The surgeon will check the quality and amount of your breast skin, and if you're considering flap reconstruction, he'll determine whether you have sufficient tissue at the donor site. You should also review his portfolio of before-and-after patient photos; this will probably reflect only his best work, so ask to see photos of not-so-good reconstructions as well, to get a broader perspective—not all surgeons are comfortable showing these or may not make them available, but it doesn't hurt to ask. Use the following tips to make the most of your limited appointment time.

Come prepared. Even the best doctor can't explain all the nuances of a procedure or recovery in a single appointment. Learn as much as you can on your own, and then make a list of the questions you would most like to have answered during the consultation. Ask questions to assess and compare the different ways surgeons approach reconstruction.

- Which reconstruction option is best for me and why?
- How many reconstructive surgeries of this type have you performed?
- How many do you do in a year?
- May I see your before-and-after patient photos with this procedure?
- May I speak with a couple of your patients who've had the same procedure?
- How will my nipple and areola be affected by my reconstruction (if you're having nipple-sparing mastectomy)?
- Will you perform the reconstruction through my mastectomy incision(s)? What other incisions will I have and where will they be made?
- How many surgeries and office visits will be required, over what period of time?
- What are the possible side effects and risks from the procedure?
- Do you recommend surgery for my opposite breast for symmetry (if you're having unilateral reconstruction)?

- How long will the surgery take and how long will I stay in the hospital?
- What will my recovery be like and how long will it take before I'm able to return to my normal routine?
- What's the best result I can expect?
- What if I'm unhappy with my results?

Bring your medical records. When you schedule an appointment, ask whether you should bring your pathology reports, mammograms, or other medical records for review. Then contact your doctor's office, hospital, or other facility to gather up everything you need.

Disclose medications, supplements, vitamins, and herbs. Your surgeon will advise which, if any, products you should discontinue and when you can resume taking them. This is very important, because some may interfere with circulation or healing. Include all prescribed and over-the-counter items. If you have several items to disclose, it's easier to hand your surgeon a list (table 18.1).

Don't be afraid to communicate. The most successful consultation is interactive. Describe what you want from reconstruction and voice your concerns. If you would like smaller, larger, or rounder breasts, now is the time to say so. Don't be afraid to speak up if you need something explained, spelled, or repeated. Ask your surgeon to draw you a picture to

TABLE 18.1. Sample list of medications, supplements, vitamins, and herbs to report to your doctor before surgery

Medication	Dose	Frequency	Reason
Premarin	0.625 mg	Daily	Replace hormones
Simvastatin	20 mg	Daily	Manage cholesterol
Fish oil	1,200 mg	Daily	Manage cholesterol
Black cohosh	370 mg	Daily	Reduce hot flashes
Desonide	—	As needed	Eczema
Multivitamin		Daily	Aid nutritional health

clarify a procedure. Inquire about anything that concerns or confuses you, no matter how silly or insignificant it may seem.

Take notes. Experts say we forget 50 percent of what we hear in a doctor's office. That's not surprising, because new information and terms can be overwhelming, especially when you're still dealing with treatment issues and trying to get used to the idea of mastectomy. Jot down or record the key points of your discussion so you can review them later. Better yet, bring someone with you. Four ears are better than two—your appointment buddy can take notes while you focus on listening. If you go to your appointment alone, use a tape recorder to capture your conversation with the surgeon.

Let it all sink in. Never feel pressured to make a decision about a surgeon or to schedule a procedure before you leave the office. Take time to let everything sink in and to think about what you've heard. Discuss your options with your partner or an impartial trusted friend to get another perspective.

The Value of a Second (or Third) Opinion

No single method of reconstruction is right for every woman. There are many techniques, many options, and many opinions. Reconstruction recommendations vary widely, depending on the plastic surgeon's area of expertise and preference. You have nothing to lose and everything to gain by getting a second, if not a third, opinion. Contact your health insurance company to determine under what conditions additional consultation appointments are covered. (Most health care insurance will pay for a second opinion.) Waiting for another opinion shouldn't offend a surgeon; it's standard practice with any operation.

Another opinion is always a good idea, and it can be especially helpful if you're unsure or confused about how to proceed or if you want to consider another surgeon's approach and recommendation. You may end up choosing the first surgeon you speak with, but it's good to consider other ideas. Some women feel that female surgeons are more sympathetic and can relate to reconstruction issues better than men can. Women who are happy with their male plastic surgeons might disagree. It's best to evaluate each surgeon on his or her own merits—you are the judge of what's best for you. Remember, you're doing the hiring. You needn't feel compelled or coerced to have one surgeon or another do your surgery. If you're uncomfortable with a surgeon for any reason, find someone else. Keep looking until you find your Dr. Right.

> *After much research and window shopping with each and every consultation, I found a plastic surgeon who was the perfect match for me in every sense. I was immediately struck by his casual demeanor and appreciated his reassurances, availability, track record, and references; yet, it was his striking confidence that won me over. We reviewed many of his before-and-after pictures to gain a real sense of what I wanted. We discussed the expander method at great lengths and mutually felt this route would provide optimal reconstruction for me. He was there for all of my medical needs and always returned my phone calls and e-mails promptly. Most of all, he was an absolute perfectionist and I appreciated his artistic abilities.* —Marie

Tips for Travelers

You're fortunate if you live in a city with experienced reconstructive surgeons. But the best reconstructive opportunities aren't always possible locally, particularly if you live in a small town or rural area. If the surgeons and techniques you want aren't available nearby, you'll need to decide whether you'll settle for the local expertise or travel for your reconstruction. Even though journeying to another city for your surgery involves more time, effort, and cost—insurance doesn't typically pay for travel and hotel costs, and your out-of-pocket expense may be higher—if you're able to do so, it may be worthwhile to pack up for a few days to get the surgeon and procedure you want. Many reconstructive surgery practices, especially those that practice breast reconstruction exclusively, have patient relations coordinators who can facilitate consultation appointments, coordinate insurance coverage, and recommend nearby hotels that provide patient discounts. If you're having immediate reconstruction, they'll also recommend a breast surgeon with whom they work, so you won't need to search for someone to do your mastectomy. If you can manage it, you can drive or fly in for a consultation and return home the same day. If that doesn't work, many surgeons offer distant consults: you can swap information and provide photos of your breasts and donor site by e-mail or video conference. If you like what you hear, you can then arrange an in-person consultation or schedule your surgery. Once your surgery date is on the calendar, you can complete all the necessary pre-op testing in your hometown, with a copy of the results forwarded to your distant plastic surgeon. As a precaution, you should contact a local plastic surgeon or surgical oncologist before your reconstruction to ask whether they'll provide follow-up care if you need it.

It may be hard to fathom traveling far from home to have surgery and all that this entails, but many women do. Your surgeon's office will advise you of the necessary travel requirements. Generally, you'll need to be away from home for about a week: you'll have a pre-op appointment on the day before your surgery, and then stay overnight in the hospital for implant surgery or three to five days after flap surgery. After you're discharged, you'll need to remain in town (with family or friends or in a hotel) until your post-op appointment or until your surgeon clears you to return home. If you'll be flying home after a flap reconstruction, arranging for a wheelchair at the airport will avoid long walks through the terminal and jostling crowds, and you'll be able to pre-board the airplane. Ask your surgeon to provide a copy of your operative report and a letter stating that you have surgical drains, just in case you're questioned by airport security. If you have tissue expanders with metal valves (they may set off security scanners) carry the Device Information Card provided by your surgeon. You may still be subject to a secondary screening.

I did an enormous amount of research until I found the procedure and doctors that I felt were the best fit for me, which meant traveling about four hours from my home for surgery. I knew recovery would be uncomfortable, and rather than having to do the four-hour drive multiple times, I opted to recover in a hotel. By being away from home I was forced to take it easy, which would never have happened at home, and I was able to truly relax and recover. —Jess

CHAPTER NINETEEN

Paying for Your Reconstruction

*My in-network surgeons performed the procedure I wanted,
and I didn't give it a second thought. I never even saw a bill,
so I assume everything was paid.*　　　　　—DAWN

If you've had a smooth relationship with your insurance company while
dealing with breast cancer or other serious health issues, you're among the
fortunate. Paying for your reconstruction is often not straightforward,
even when you have insurance coverage. While numerous women have
absolutely no problems at all with reconstruction-related insurance coverage, too many say that dealing with their insurers is almost as nerve-
wracking as coping with the diagnosis or the surgery.

The Women's Health and Cancer Rights Act (1998) applies to individual health policies and group health plans of employers and unions. (Certain church plans and government plans are excluded.) The law requires
insurers that pay for mastectomy related to breast cancer or any medical condition to also cover prostheses and reconstructive procedures
(table 19.1). Also known as Janet's Law, the legislation is named after
Janet Franquet, a woman who was denied reconstructive surgery after mastectomy because her insurance company considered replacement of a
breast to be cosmetic and medically unnecessary. Her surgeon generously
reconstructed her breast for free. Franquet pursued a lengthy appeals
process, which she eventually won.

The WHCRA recognizes breast reconstruction as more than cosmetic
surgery, but it stops short of guaranteeing your absolute choice in the
matter—it doesn't set payment rates or guarantee payment for specific
procedures, surgeons, or hospitals. Although the law doesn't extend to
Medicare and Medicaid, both programs cover the cost of prostheses and
reconstructive surgery. To learn more about the law, search for "WHCRA"
at the Department of Labor's Employee Benefits Security Administration

TABLE 19.1. Requirements and limits of the Women's Health and Cancer Rights Act

Requires insurers to cover:	Does *not*:
Certain services relating to mastectomy as determined by you and your surgeon	Require insurance companies to pay for mastectomy
Breast prostheses and special mastectomy bras	Set payment rates, or guarantee specific procedures, surgeons, or hospitals
All stages of immediate and delayed breast reconstruction*	Apply to all plans; certain government, school, and church plans are exempt (some cover mastectomy and reconstruction anyway)
Additional procedures to achieve symmetry, including modification of the healthy breast after unilateral reconstruction	Provide retroactive coverage; if you weren't insured with your current plan before January 1999 or you had your mastectomy before that time, your current insurer isn't obligated to cover your reconstruction now
Treatment for lymphedema and other complications related to mastectomy or reconstruction	

*If you change insurance companies and your new plan covers mastectomy, it must also cover reconstruction.

website (www.askebsa.dol.gov). The ASPS website (www.plasticsurgery .org) provides links to state laws (search for "state laws on breast reconstruction").

The Affordable Care Act of 2010 prohibits health insurers from imposing lifetime dollar limits on annual caps, limiting essential benefits, or excluding individuals or canceling their policies based on pre-existing health conditions, including breast cancer. Plans that cover mastectomy and reconstruction must include a description of these benefits in the Summary of Benefits and Coverage provided annually to the insured. (Some policies and plans that were issued on or before March 23, 2010, are grandfathered and don't have to comply with some provisions of the law. These grandfathered plans may not impose lifetime benefit caps or arbitrarily cancel coverage. However, they may impose annual benefit caps and exclude individuals for pre-existing conditions.)

Most states also have laws regarding mastectomy and breast reconstruction. Some mandate minimum hospital stays, while others provide additional protection beyond WHCRA. Your state health insurance agency or insurance commissioner can also provide more information.

Are You Covered?

Dealing proactively with your insurance company before your surgery is a smart move that most likely will avoid unpleasant payment surprises. Never assume your health insurance will automatically cover your reconstruction. Check your benefits handbook, plan document, or policy to determine what is covered and what isn't. Call the customer service department if you need further clarification. Your most valuable ally is the insurance specialist in your plastic surgeon's office. While the insurance experience may be new to you, she deals with preauthorizations, payments, denials, and related issues every day and has probably already had experience dealing with your insurance company. She'll be familiar with the appropriate codes that insurance carriers require for each and every service, and will help you to navigate the insurance maze and do much of the footwork to arrange payment with your insurer.

Questions for your health insurance company:

- Does my plan cover mastectomy? (If the answer is yes, it must also cover reconstruction.)
- How many "second" opinions are covered?
- How should I obtain preauthorization for my surgery?
- Am I limited to in-network surgeons and services?
- If I travel to another surgeon who specializes in a particular technique not available within my network, what expenses will be covered?
- What are my total out-of-pocket costs if I go to an out-of-network surgeon? (This is primarily a question for your plastic surgeon, but

asking this of your insurer will give you an idea of what is covered and what is not.)

- Is there a limit to the amount of coverage provided?
- Is my hospital stay covered? If so, for how many days?
- Are the other health care professionals involved in my surgery also covered?
- Will all payments be made directly to providers?

How much will you have to pay? Without a standard fee structure, costs for mastectomy and reconstruction vary widely, depending on where your surgeon practices and the procedure you choose: the cost of an implant or DIEP reconstruction in New York may be quite different from the cost for the same procedures in San Diego or Des Moines.

Like all businesses, health care insurers limit services to control costs and increase profits. Their fee schedule is generally based on what they consider to be "usual and customary" charges for the geographical area, but this is often only a fraction of a surgeon's "sticker price."

Working within your health plan. If your health plan covers mastectomy and reconstruction, it must do so under its overall guidelines. You still have to pay any *deductibles* and *co-payments* routinely required for other plan benefits. In other words, if your plan normally pays 80 percent of medical services and you pay the remaining 20 percent, the same schedule applies to your reconstructive expenses. Be sure to follow your plan's process for requesting reconstruction, including preauthorization.

The rules of your health plan also apply to your mastectomy and reconstruction. If your plan generally only pays for services with *in-network* physicians, the same applies to breast and plastic surgeons. If you have this type of policy, choosing one of these preapproved surgeons will be to your financial advantage and will limit your *out-of-pocket costs* to whatever deductible and co-pay for which you are ordinarily responsible. In-network providers agree to accept predetermined fees for services they provide. This is usually much less than their customary fees—they write off the remaining unpaid balance. Your plan may limit your choice of surgeons to those who practice locally, or it may include surgeons in other cities or states.

Out-of-network providers don't have payment agreements with the insurer and aren't as likely to write off a balance due. That translates into higher out-of-pocket costs for you. A surgeon may accept a combination of your insurer's offered payment and your co-pay as payment in full. If he does not, you may be responsible for the balance to make up the difference. It's important to determine your total out-of-pocket expenses before you schedule surgery. If your surgeon doesn't accept your insurance and advises you to pay in advance and then seek reimbursement from your health insurer, realize your financial risk: your insurance company may compensate you for only a small part of the amount you paid, or none at all.

You may deduct a percentage of your total out-of-pocket medical expenses from your state and federal income taxes, including costs related to your breast cancer treatment and reconstruction and other health-related expenses you pay during the tax year. Check with your tax professional or see IRS Publication 502 for a complete list of deductible expenses.

Appealing When the Answer Is No

Several days after your preauthorization request, a letter arrives from your insurance company. You're expecting an approval, but find a refusal instead: your request has been denied. Angry, frustrated, and feeling helpless, women often give up at this point. Is it worth the effort to challenge your insurance company's decision? Yes! You have nothing to lose and so much to gain. Despite federal and state laws protecting a woman's right to breast reconstruction, denials occur more frequently than you might imagine. The Affordable Care Act protects your right to appeal health care denials. If you feel strongly about overturning your denial, you must act as your own advocate. You should know before you begin that attempting to get your insurer to recant can be frustrating and time consuming. But health care organizations aren't perfect—they make mistakes; nor are they invincible. Other women have won appeals, and you may be able to do the same, depending on the circumstances. And here's a little secret: often simply appealing the decision gets it overturned—more than half of all Medicare and health plan denials in California, for example, are overturned when they are appealed. Your own Department of Health can provide statistics for the state where you live. Denials are often the result of administrative error at the insurance company. The health insurer may receive incorrect codes from a billing physician or be unclear or mistaken about why your service was necessary. If the company realizes it's made a mistake or feels it's more cost effective to grant your request than fight it, you'll likely win your appeal.

Your health insurance company must state the reason for refusal in its notification to you. It may be difficult to find rhyme or reason for the logic behind the decision, but all health insurance policies are different and coverage varies, depending on many variables. You're least likely to encounter problems when you choose an in-network surgeon who provides traditional implant, lat flap, TRAM or DIEP flap reconstruction. Requests for newer procedures and out-of-network services are more likely to be refused. Here's how to go about appealing a denial.

Follow the process. Challenging a denial is your legal right. If you're going to appeal, you must follow exactly your plan's appeal procedure as it is described in your denial letter and your benefits manual. The process will involve internal appeals handled by your insurance company. By law, employer-provided insurance plans may have no more than two appeal levels. At the first level, appeals are typically decided by a claims reviewer and signed off by a medical professional; a denial is least likely to be over-turned at this level. The second appeal is considered by a review panel that includes at least one physician in the same specialty you requested— in this case, plastic surgery. If your insurance carrier allows it, try an in-person appeal at this level, which can be more effective than a written appeal. Submit all paperwork on time to meet the deadlines for each level of appeal—if your policy states you have 30 days to appeal a decision, work diligently to comply. Send your appeal by certified mail to the appropri-ate contact listed in your denial letter.

Focus on the reason for denial. Call your insurance company and re-quest a copy of the medical opinion on which your denial is based; this should be the focus of your request for reconsideration. Also, request a case manager for your appeal. She'll become familiar with your case, and contacting her directly will save you the time and hassle of having to go through customer service representatives each time you call. In most cases, your denial will be based on one of the following reasons:

- "Benefit not provided" means your plan doesn't provide the service you requested. Check your benefits summary to see whether mastectomy is a covered benefit. If it is, the insurer must also provide coverage for reconstruction. Include a copy of the WHCRA with your appeal letter, stating that the denial appears to be in violation of the law.
- "Not medically necessary" is one of the most common reasons for denial. It means that the insurer doesn't consider your procedure to be necessary for your continued good health. If your insurer vetoes your request for prophylactic mastectomy, for example, ask your oncologist, primary care physician, or medical geneticist (or all three) to write letters describing your family history of breast cancer and confirming your high-risk status. Attach studies showing that prophylactic bilateral mastectomy is an effective and accepted risk management protocol for high-risk women. In some cases, the rejection may be a result of a simple administrative error. If your surgeon's office uses the wrong billing code and description when submitting a claim to your insurer, the problem can be resolved by resubmitting with the correct codes. If you're trying to improve symmetry by changing your implant to a larger size, for example, your insurer is likely to reject "patient prefers increased breast size" or "exchange 300 cc breast implant to 400 cc breast implant" as the reason for the procedure. You're more likely to gain approval when the description clearly states that the revision surgery is necessary to improve asymmetry or other problems caused by mastectomy or breast reconstruction. If your plastic surgeon routinely performs breast reconstruction, his billing specialist will be familiar with what needs to be submitted. But it's always a good idea to check when you receive a denial.
- "Out-of-network" is a common reason for rejecting a reconstruction request and one of the most difficult appeals to win, especially if in-network surgeons provide the procedure you want. Unless you can show that your request is medically necessary, you're not likely to have a denial for out-of-network benefits reversed. Your insurer will most

likely refuse your request to go to a surgeon who doesn't belong to your insurer's physician network for your TUG reconstruction, for instance, if an in-network surgeon also provides the same procedure. However, if TUG is the only procedure for which you're a candidate (perhaps your implants failed after radiation and you're too thin for any other flap reconstruction) and no in-network surgeons perform TUG, you have a stronger argument. If you can obtain documentation from an in-network surgeon validating your decision, so much the better.

- "Procedure is experimental" means your carrier doesn't recognize or accept the procedure you requested. The company may be unfamiliar with a particular type of reconstruction, and once educated, might reverse its denial. This may be the case if you prefer DIEP, GAP, direct-to-implant, or other newer reconstructive procedures that your carrier considers to be above and beyond the more traditional tissue expansion, lat flaps, and TRAM. As more women have these procedures, this type of denial will hopefully become less frequent. Support your case with peer-reviewed studies and articles in medical journals that prove your requested procedure is established, bona fide, and safe. If your insurance carrier turns down your request for a DIEP reconstruction because in-network surgeons already provide TRAM procedures, point out the shorter hospital stay and fewer postoperative complications with DIEP. Cite Johns Hopkins Hospital, one of the most respected medical cancer facilities in the world, which no longer offers pedicled TRAM surgeries because it considers DIEP to be far superior. (Search for "reconstructive breast surgery options" at www.hopkinsmedicine.org for supporting documentation to include in your appeal.) One other circumstance may work in your favor: if you can show that other insurers cover the procedure you want (your surgeon's billing coordinator can help with this), you may sway the company to change its opinion and, in doing so, help yourself and pave the way for other women who request the procedure in the future.

Unfortunately, my insurance company is really dragging its corporate feet and has not yet authorized my PBM. Their "BRCA expert" seems very ill-informed so I am trying to look at this as an educational opportunity for them. If I cannot prevail, I will change to a new insurer in January. —*Samantha*

Build your case. The hardest part of an appeal is crafting your response without letting your frustration and emotions get in the way. Although your reconstruction is a very personal matter for you, it's a business decision for your insurance company. And while it is disheartening to have your request refused, this is the time for logic to prevail. Resist the temptation to sit down and fire off an immediate angry response. Be aggressively persistent without being hostile. You have a better chance of succeeding if your appeal is brief and clear and includes fact-based evidence that clearly justifies your argument. Don't waste your time reiterating what the insurer already knows. Stick to the issue at hand, focusing on evidence that refutes the reason for rejection. Your plastic surgeon's office may provide sample letters that have worked successfully for other patients.

Start working on your appeal strategy soon after you receive notification of denial. Gather up all the information you need: applicable medical records, supporting letters from physicians, and research materials that help make your case. Top it off with a formal cover letter that includes the following:

- your insurance policy number
- acknowledgment that you've received the denial
- your appeal claim number
- a request for a "physician review," which means your appeal will be reviewed by a plastic surgeon
- a request for reconsideration

It doesn't hurt to ask your case manager to arrange a call between your plastic surgeon and the medical director who will be reviewing your appeal. (When surgeons actually speak together, you may have a greater chance of having your denial overturned.) Send copies of the entire package to your physician and your lawyer, if you have one, and a copy to your state legislator (the latter probably won't help, but it can't hurt).

Ask for help. Don't be shy about asking your physicians to provide supportive letters or point you in the right direction for peer-reviewed studies and medical reports on the procedure you want. You can also search PubMed.gov, the U.S. National Library of Medicine's online repository of medical studies. The nonprofit Patient Advocate Foundation (www .patientadvocate.org) will help you along the way, at no charge, and act as a liaison between you and your insurance company—the organization's website also has sample appeal letters. Livestrong (https://www.livestrong .org/we-can-help/livestrong-navigation) is another helpful resource.

Keep a paper trail. Keep copies of all written correspondence and a call log of your conversations with insurance company employees, noting the date, time, details of the discussion, and name of the employee. If a discrepancy comes up, you'll have supportive documentation.

When All Else Fails

Once you've exhausted your insurer's appeals process (but not before), you can request an appeal with an external reviewer at the state level. This secondary appeal is conducted by an independent medical review board of plastic surgeons who are empowered to sustain or overrule an insurance company's decision—the insurer's denial will probably be upheld if the panel finds it conforms to state law and abides by the company's stated rules of coverage. The verdict may take 30 to 60 days; you can request an expedited decision if you show sufficient cause (such as your imminent mastectomy due to an aggressive breast cancer) for an emergency ruling.

Your appeal rights may vary, depending on the type of health insurance plan you have and the process required by the state in which you live. Fully insured plans (in which your employer buys health coverage from an insurance company) are regulated by state laws, so any external appeal process is administered by the state. Self-insured plans (your employer pays claims from its own resources, even if it contracts with an insurance company to administer the plan) are governed by the Employee Retirement Income Security Act (ERISA), a federal law; these plans aren't required to comply with all state laws. Therefore, if your plan is self-insured, you may have no appeal rights at the state level. You can learn more about state and federal insurance laws and find information about appeals at the U.S. Department of Health and Human Services website (www.healthcare .gov). Check with your state's department of insurance to learn more about the appeal process. Find contact information for your state at the National Insurance Commission's website (www.naic.org/state_web_map.htm).

The Affordable Care Act mandates impartial internal and external appeal processes for everyone who is covered by a plan that was created after March 23, 2010. States must provide independent, impartial reviewers who meet certain standards, keep written records, and aren't affected by conflicts of interest. If you're not protected by state law, you can appeal to a federal external review program. If the external reviewer agrees with your appeal, your health care plan must pay for the benefit in question. If your insurance company's denial is upheld, your only other option is to pursue legal action. It may be worth the money to pay for an hour's consultation with a health insurance lawyer to determine applicable fees, success with similar appeals, and whether she thinks you have a case. If you can't afford the fee, contact the Patient Advocate Foundation or your state bar association to inquire about lawyers who will write an appeal letter for you at no charge. Contact your state legislator or insurance commissioner if you feel you're being treated unfairly or illegally.

Help for the uninsured. Reconstruction can be expensive, and for most women, it's cost prohibitive without insurance or financial assistance. If you don't have health insurance and you can't afford mastectomy and reconstruction, you may be eligible for programs for low-income and uninsured women. Contact your local medical center, teaching facility, or ACS branch office to see whether they're aware of special local funding programs or know of plastic surgeons who donate reconstructive services for a few women each year (many surgeons do). My Hope Chest (www.myhopechest.org), the United Breast Cancer Foundation (www .ubcf.org), and other charitable breast cancer organizations may offer financial help for your surgery. If paying out of pocket is your only alternative, many surgeons offer reduced fees and payment schedules for breast cancer survivors. CareCredit (www.carecredit.com) offers payment plans for medical services, including breast reconstruction, for as long as 60 months.

My insurance company was great. My benefits manual outlined how mastectomy and reconstruction were covered. My in-network surgeons performed the procedure I wanted, and I didn't give it a second thought. I never even saw a bill, so I assume everything was paid. —Dawn

I was told by my insurance company's customer service department that PBM wasn't covered under any circumstances. I was so angry, I stomped into my boss's office and told her I thought it was incredibly unfair. She contacted our human resources director, who arranged a call for me with a manager at the insurance company. When I explained my BRCA status, the manager said that sometimes the customer service personnel made mistakes and assured me that my PBM would be covered. It was a good thing I pursued this, because my PBM and reconstruction were both paid for without problems. —Judy

After seeing my friend's fabulous reconstruction results, I was determined to go to her plastic surgeon, who happened to be in another state and was out-of-network for me, but my health insurance company denied my request. Even though I spent hours talking with people at the insurance company and writing appeals, I couldn't get them to change their minds. —Trish

Other Types of Insurance

If you work for a company with 50 or more employees, the Family Medical Leave Act (www.dol.gov, search for "FMLA") provides 12 weeks of unpaid, job-protected medical leave for "a serious health condition that makes the employee unable to perform the essential functions of his or her job." (You can also break up the 12 weeks into smaller increments, such as taking off every other Friday to recover from your expander fills.) You must have worked for the employer for at least 1,250 hours in the previous 12 months at a location where at least 50 employees are employed or within 75 miles of the location. If you take FMLA leave, your employer must provide full health benefits while you're away from the job and restore you to your previous position or a similar job with the same salary and benefits when you return.

If you have a short-term disability plan before your surgery, it will work like an insurance plan for your wages: depending on the amount of your premium and the terms of your policy, the policy pays you a portion or all of your regular work pay while you're unable to return to work.

CHAPTER TWENTY

Making Difficult Decisions

You do as much research as you can by reading and talking to people who have the appropriate knowledge and experience; then you do what's right for you. —JILL

You may have a team of family, friends, soul sisters, and medical professionals supporting your pending mastectomy and reconstruction, but guess who most influences your decisions?

You do.

Reconstruction can be an exciting and terrifying possibility. The decisions you face are complicated and intensely personal, and no one can make them for you. With mastectomy looming ahead, you may know precisely how you want to proceed. More likely, you're living in a state of uncertainty about what to do and when to do it. Should you have reconstruction? Is nipple-sparing mastectomy an option you would like to pursue? Would implants or a tissue flap give you a better result? Should you travel for a procedure you can't have locally or for a more experienced surgeon who can offer you a better reconstructive outcome? Making your own informed decisions about reconstruction can help restore the lack of control you may feel during your diagnosis and treatment. So how do you find answers when you're not even sure of the right questions?

Ten Steps in the Right Direction

Making the best personal decisions may seem like a tall order, considering the many procedures and options you need to learn about and sort through. With so much to absorb, you may feel you're stuck on a merry-go-round of endless terms and concepts. The following tips will help you make your way through the onslaught of information and what-ifs in front of you.

1. *Establish a positive attitude.* Think of your research as an empowering action rather than an awful chore. Your investigative efforts will help you make a confident decision.

2. *Take time to learn.* When it comes to surgery, informed is always better than impetuous. Knowing about the benefits and limitations of various reconstructive options gives you something special: the power of choice. It's never too early to start researching your post-mastectomy options. Breast cancer isn't a medical emergency for most women, and you needn't make a decision that you haven't had time to consider thoroughly. Unless you've been diagnosed with an aggressive breast cancer, taking two to three weeks to learn about reconstruction probably won't adversely affect your health. You should, of course, discuss this research interval with your medical team. If you're having preventive mastectomy, you have the luxury of time to consider reconstruction. You would probably compare loan rates before financing a home, and get to know someone pretty well before marrying them or forming a business partnership—it's only logical to approach a decision concerning your physical and emotional well-being with the same scrutiny. To use a corny football analogy, don't sit on the bench. Suit up and get in the game. Be your own advocate.

3. *Recruit a study buddy.* Having a research helper saves time and provides a second perspective. Your spouse or partner may be the best person for the task; sharing the experience can help to build understanding, commitment, and compassion. If this isn't practical, ask a relative or close friend to assist you.

4. *Be patient and persistent.* Take things one step at a time. Don't let frustration get you down. When you think you can't absorb any more information (but need to), take a break. Have lunch with a friend, play with your kids, get lost in a novel, or go for a walk.

5. *Deal with data.* Always use credible information sources. As much as possible, weed out the influences of media hype, personal anecdote, and urban myth. Make your decisions based on the facts of a particular procedure and a surgeon's expertise.

6. *Know when to stop.* At some point, you need to assess all the data you've gathered and make your decision. If you're still unsure, consider whether it's best to delay your reconstruction.

7. Sort through your options. When you first learn that mastectomy is a certainty, you may already have a particular reconstruction procedure in mind. Even so, it's still wise to consider all the possibilities available to you. Understanding your options will demystify reconstruction, replacing the unknown with the expected, and reducing your anxiety about the various ways your breasts can be rebuilt. Along the way, you may discover that reconstruction can give you better breasts than you expected, or you may find that it requires more than you're willing to go through.

8. Take time to absorb. Even after you make the decision to have reconstruction, you may still have doubts about the procedure. It's not unusual to feel this way. Experts say shock, denial, anger, and depression typically come before acceptance. Meanwhile, life goes on. There's work to be done, a home to manage, perhaps kids to raise and pets to feed. Give yourself time to let everything sink in and reflect on what you've learned.

9. Prioritize your alternatives. Your choice of a particular reconstructive procedure will be influenced by many factors. Perhaps you don't want to have additional scars from a flap procedure, you don't want to risk complications with implants after radiation, or traveling to another city is not an option. Your priority might be to have the quickest reconstruction possible or the best possible results—or both. You might not be compelled to replace your breasts at all. As you consider all the variables, use a process of elimination to whittle the possibilities down to procedures that interest you and for which you are a candidate (table 20.1).

10. Make your decision. Consider the input of loved ones, physicians, and other women who have had a mastectomy, and then listen to your own instincts. Others may influence what you decide, but you're the one who must go through the surgery and recovery, and you're the one who will live with the results. It's you, after all, who best knows your body. With many options available, the tough decisions—the what, when, who, why, and how of breast reconstruction—are up to you (figure 20.1). Weigh all of the pros and cons for each procedure to choose the one you feel is best. Whatever you decide is the right choice.

TABLE 20.1. Fill-in table to assess your breast reconstruction options

Implants or flaps?	Procedure	Acceptable procedure?	Acceptable scar/recovery?	Available locally?	Sufficient donor tissue?	Insurance coverage?
Implants	Expander-to-implant					
	Hybrid expander					
	Direct-to-implant					
Tissue flaps	Latissimus dorsi (lat)					
	Attached TRAM					
	Free TRAM					
	Muscle-sparing TRAM					
	DIEP					
	SGAP/IGAP					
	TUG					
	[Other]					
BRAVA+AFT						

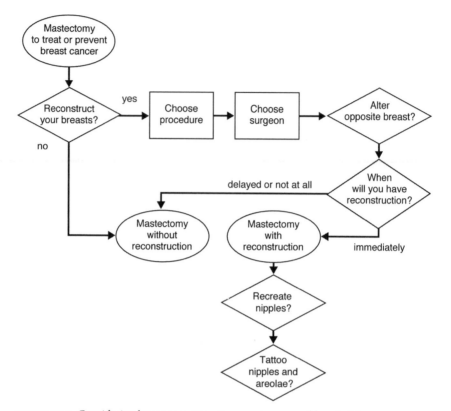

FIGURE 20.1. Considering breast reconstruction requires several key decisions.

My mother was diagnosed with breast cancer at age 45 and died five years later when I was sixteen, so my high-risk status raised a host of monsters in my head. I was initially terrified and overwhelmed by the information, and then decided quickly to have prophylactic oophorectomy and mastectomy—I did not want my two children to lose their mother as early as I did. I considered implant reconstruction, the only type available locally, but I was interested in flap reconstruction as soon as I learned about it. I was lucky to connect with someone who had already interviewed a number of the doctors in my state and nationally who do flap procedures, and to benefit from her extensive research. The more I learned about flap surgery, the more I knew it was the best choice for me. Using my own tissue for a more natural look and feel, and not having implants that would need to be replaced down the road, were the most important factors. Once I saw a friend's beautiful DIEP flap reconstruction, my fears about the surgery were greatly relieved. I know that combined with nipple-sparing mastectomy, it was the best balance of risk reduction and cosmetic result. —*Sonya*

I agonized over my reconstruction choice, but after thinking and rethinking my options, I ultimately chose implants, because I just couldn't accommodate the childcare and time away from work a flap surgery would require. —*Rachel*

Other Sources of Information and Inspiration

Not so long ago, reconstruction choices were limited and information was hard to come by. With a few clicks of your mouse, you can now bring an amazing assortment of information and personal experience directly to your desktop, if you know where to look for the bits and pieces. And it's all free. Medical reports, articles, and personal reconstruction journals await on the Internet. Before-and-after color photos of women who have had mastectomy and reconstruction can be found on websites of plastic surgeons and the American Society of Plastic Surgeons (www .plasticsurgery.org). Sorting through all this information can be overwhelming, however, and before you know it, you may have spent days in front of your computer but feel no closer to getting the answers you need. Narrow your search to specific terms. Looking for "direct-to-implant reconstruction" or "TUG flap breast reconstruction recovery," for example, will refine your search. Bookmark your favorite websites for easy return. If you're curious and have the fortitude, you can watch actual breast and nipple reconstruction operations at ORlive (www.orlive.com) and You-Tube (www.youtube.com).

Mastectomy and reconstruction used to be topics women kept to themselves. While some still prefer to keep their experiences private, many are happy to share the details of their reconstruction and recovery in person, in chat rooms, and on social networking sites such as Facebook and Twitter. Discussion groups at Susan G. Komen for the Cure (ww5.komen .org), Cancer Support Network (csn.cancer.org), and Johns Hopkins Medicine (www.hopkinsbreastcenter.org/services/ask _expert) frequently have postings related to reconstruction. The FORCE message boards (www .facingourrisk.org) are one of the most informative and supportive online neighborhoods, particularly concerning reconstruction. Members have been through every imaginable breast cancer and reconstruction experience. No matter where you are in the journey, there's a huge sisterhood of previvors and survivors with reconstruction experience who have "been there and done that" and are ready and willing to lend a virtual shoulder. Having experienced the same emotional roller coaster and confusion, they can relate to what you're feeling better than anyone else. One caveat about discussions of mastectomy and breast reconstruction on blogs and message boards: women are often passionate about their reconstruction, whether they're happy or dissatisfied with their results. Realize that someone else's experience won't necessarily be yours, and her choice may not be the best solution for you. Try not to substitute personal opinion for medical advice or use the experiences of just one or two women to make your decision.

Local support groups can also be helpful. Contact your nearest ACS office, hospital, or breast cancer center to see whether they sponsor reconstruction discussion groups, seminars, or lectures. Your library and bookstore shelves and online retailers offer memoirs of women who have gone through the same emotional upheaval that you're experiencing, including these exceptional examples:

> *In the Family* (DVD), by Joanna Rudnick, documents the 27-year-old filmmaker's experiences and conflicts dealing with the impact of a positive BRCA gene test.
>
> *Pretty Is What Changes: Impossible Choices, the Breast Cancer Gene, and How I Defied My Destiny* is an award-winning memoir by 34-year-old TV writer Jessica Queller and how she dealt with difficult decisions about her breasts when she tested positive for a BRCA mutation just 11 months after she lost her mother to ovarian cancer.
>
> *Spinning Straw into Gold: Your Emotional Recovery from Breast Cancer*, by psychotherapist and breast cancer survivor Ronnie Kaye, explains how to deal with the emotional side effects of breast cancer.
>
> *Why I Wore Lipstick to My Mastectomy*, by Geralyn Lucas, chronicles a 27-year-old woman's unusual and inspiring approach to her mastectomy and reconstruction in our beauty-obsessed culture.

CHAPTER TWENTY-ONE

Information for Family and Friends

When my wife faced mastectomy, I felt a deep and strong conviction that all I wanted was for her to make choices that would most increase her chances of survival, and I would support the decisions she made. —DAN

If someone you care about is facing mastectomy, breast reconstruction, or both, your support will be a welcome gift. Surgery and recovery can be difficult roads to walk alone, and while you can't go through the experience for her, you can rally to her side, providing love and strength to see her through.

Hints for Family Members

For parents. It's difficult to see your daughter struggle with life-altering decisions, pain, and anxiety, especially if you've faced a similar situation yourself. You would probably be willing to trade places and spare her the experience if you could. You can help in the weeks before surgery, which can be nerve-wracking for her. Join in as she researches mastectomy and reconstruction. Read through this book so you'll know what to expect. Help her put her house in order before surgery and arrange to get things done during her recovery. Most important, help by supporting whatever decisions she makes about mastectomy and reconstruction, even if you disagree. Understand that even though these surgeries aren't life threatening, they require sacrifice and recovery.

For siblings. Now is the time to support your sister, whether you live down the street or across the country. It's not the best time to bring up family grudges or disagreements, but it's the perfect time to let your words or deeds show that you care. Call frequently to make her laugh when she's down. Buy her a pair of pretty pajamas (button in the front) or something that will comfort her in the hospital and when she returns home. Bring or send her a teddy bear, flowers, or a balloon bouquet. If she's a mom, shift your schedule to care for your nieces and nephews. Take them to school, the zoo, or the movies. Attend their sports activities when your sister cannot. Be supportive; stay in touch to express your good thoughts and encouragement.

Food for Thought for Partners and Spouses

Mastectomy and reconstruction are feared events that you hoped you'd never have to face. But now you do. Unless you've experienced a loved one's surgery and recovery, you may be overwhelmed and scared, and you may feel clueless about how you can best help her. This may be frustrating for you, particularly if your usual approach to problems is to try to fix them. You can't fix this situation—you can't change the fact that she needs a mastectomy and you can't shorten her recovery—you can do many things to help her as she goes through the experience.

Be her sounding board. An old saying goes, "God gave us two ears but only one mouth. Some people say that's because he wanted us to spend twice as much time listening as talking." Listening is a skill, and now, more than ever, your mate will appreciate your sympathetic ear. Give her your full attention as she expresses her concerns and asks your opinion about the many "ifs" involved in reconstruction decisions. Listen to her fears, issues, and questions with an open mind. Consider why she wants to travel to a distant city for reconstruction when there are plastic surgeons in your hometown or why she's leaning in favor of tissue flap reconstruction when implants would be quicker. You don't have to—and shouldn't—make decisions for her, but it will be a comfort for her to share ideas with you and know she can confide in you.

Be her partner. You may not be able to rescue your partner, but you can join her on the journey. Let her know that you're there for her, and that the two of you will go through this life-changing experience together. Be an extra set of ears at her doctor's appointments—ask questions, take notes, and look at before-and-after patient photos together. Then discuss what you've learned when you get home. Learn with her about reconstructive options and what to expect from recovery, so that you can approach these issues as a team. Search the Internet for helpful articles, and then print them out so you can read and discuss them together. While she's recovering, arrange (and rearrange) pillows so she can rest comfortably. Maybe a gentle back or foot rub would be just the ticket. Run interference with friends who call to see how she's doing, and make sure the kids don't jump up on Mommy. Learn how to empty her drains. Your attentiveness will be immensely reassuring. Comfort her if she needs to have a good cry or to just vent about what she's having to endure. Take time to read *Breast Cancer Husband* by Marc Silver, a revealing look into how a woman's surgery and recovery affects her partner, and tips for coping with the experience.

Be her communicator. Say yes when friends ask whether they can help. Coordinate a brigade to deliver meals, walk the dog, run errands, and shuttle the kids to school and activities. Send e-mail status reports to family and friends, so you won't be inundated with calls to check on the patient. Use CaringBridge (www.caringbridge.com) or other social networking sites to stay connected.

Be her cheerleader. Although most women return to their pre-surgery lives after mastectomy and reconstruction without additional problems, the road to recovery is sometimes littered with setbacks. Impatient to have recovery over and done with, your partner may be fragile, fatigued, and anxious. A small roadblock can seem enormous. Respect her feelings when she's disappointed because her drains need to remain a while longer. Understand when she's not upbeat because her expanders are uncomfortable or she is coping with an infection. Listen to her concerns and let her know that although these things feel devastating now, they can be corrected and will get better. Reassure her if she's disappointed with how her new breasts look. Remind her to give reconstruction adequate time to improve, and support her if she wants to pursue corrective action. Let her talk when she feels like it, and support her need for silence when she doesn't. Be there for her, whether she's angry, impatient, or scared. Be generous with gentle hugs when she is overwhelmed or frustrated.

Be her lover. Some women have no problem at all with the transition back to a normal sex life after reconstruction, while others feel irreparably changed. Be patient if your partner's ordeal has left her nervous about intimacy; she may feel insecure about her breasts or how she looks. Use actions and words to reassure her that mastectomy and reconstruction are not the end of your sex life together. Tell her that you still desire her and still consider her whole—these are powerful, reassuring words at a time when she may question her own femininity. Read the section "Dating, Intimacy, and Sex" in chapter 17.

Your partner needs to heal physically and emotionally. She may have trouble with one or the other, or both. Realize that while her new breast might feel the same to you, it won't be the same to her. She won't have the sensation she's used to in much of her reconstructed breast, including her nipples; she'll be unable to feel your touch—that may change some aspects of your intimacy. Encourage her to talk about how she feels, and approach troublesome issues together. Don't be afraid to include her breasts in your lovemaking; focus on the areas where she has the most feeling.

> *When my wife faced mastectomy, I felt a deep and strong conviction that all I wanted was for her to make choices that would most increase her chances of survival, and I would support the decisions she made. Although I knew that I loved her with or without breasts, I was glad that she decided to have reconstruction because I thought it would be important for her self-image. When the reconstruction was new, I felt her grief when she had no sensation and said that it felt strange when I touched her breasts. I wanted to caress them because they were a part of her; however, I quickly learned to first stroke around and between her breasts where she had feeling before touching the area that lacked sensation. In this way, we were both able to appreciate a new intimacy that included her reconstructed chest. Now, thirteen years later, I rarely think about the fact that her breasts aren't natural. She has since gained some increased sensation and that is positive for us both.   —Dan*

Issues for Caregivers

Whether family member, partner, or friend, if you're acting as a caregiver to someone who is recovering from mastectomy or reconstruction, it helps to understand the scope of her recovery and to know what to expect. Be ready to respond to whatever she needs: cold packs to reduce swelling, a sympathetic ear, or a comforting cup of tea. Help her in and out of bed. Be supportive if she has setbacks or complications. Remain calm and patient, particularly if she is used to being independent. She may need help getting into the shower or tub, for example, but she may not like asking for help. Be patient if she is abrupt because she's uncomfortable, worried, or frustrated.

If you'll be your mate's primary caregiver, you'll be dealing with two powerful sets of emotions: yours and hers. Being a caregiver can exact its own toll; it's important to balance providing support to her and supporting yourself. Keep the end target in mind: her recovery will one day be over. At times, that may be hard for both of you to keep in perspective. Meanwhile, take care of yourself, because the stress and anxiety you feel can easily undermine your own health. Eat well, get plenty of rest, and allow yourself to get away for short periods to renew your strength and spirit. Ask a relative or close friend to spend the morning with your partner while you head to the office for a few hours, or go for a walk while she has a nap. If you feel stressed, find an outlet for your emotions, especially if you're the strong silent type and it's difficult to talk about your feelings. Speak to another family member, a trusted friend, a clergyperson, or a counselor at your local cancer center. Support groups for partners of cancer survivors, including the National Alliance of Caregiving (www.caregiving .org), can be helpful. Writing about your feelings is also cathartic.

Dos and Don'ts for Friends

As we all know, actions speak louder than words; besides being practical, actions are a meaningful way to show your feelings, especially if you feel uncomfortable talking about cancer, surgery, or recovery.

Deliver meals. No matter what type of reconstruction your friend has had, she won't be spending time in the kitchen anytime soon. One of the most helpful things you can do is to deliver meals that are easily reheated— and offer to recruit neighbors and friends for meal delivery, if that hasn't already been done. A hearty soup or stew, pasta, or other main course with a salad and a dessert will be appreciated by the patient and her entire family. It's always nice to throw in extra surprises, like a funny card, cute napkins, or treats for her family or her pets.

Babysit. If the patient has children, take them out for an afternoon or stay with them during the day to ensure Mom gets her rest. Invite them over for a sleepover with your kids. Take them to school, soccer practice, play dates, and music lessons.

Run errands. During recovery, everyday errands and chores that keep a home running smoothly will slide to a halt unless someone else does them. Ask if you can do grocery shopping. Stocking your friend's kitchen with grocery essentials the day before she arrives home from the hospital will be a great help. Drop off and pick up dry cleaning, mow the lawn, or walk the dog (maybe even keep the pooch at your house until your friend recovers). Even if your help isn't initially needed, offer again in a few days.

Entertain and amuse. Recovery can be boring between naps. Drop off DVDs, magazines, crossword puzzles, Sudoku, and audio books by her favorite author. Send flowers or deliver fresh-cut bouquets from your garden. Perhaps nothing lifts the spirits as much as inspiring words. Your friend will appreciate that you took the time to send e-mails and text messages, and even the most committed technophile enjoys receiving a card in the mail—she can reread your friendly words whenever she needs a pick-me-up. Don't be afraid to send something humorous; it's good medicine.

Offer positive support. Unless you've lost your breasts and then had them rebuilt, there's no way to understand the full impact and intense emotions that go along with the experience. Consider the following guidelines to make sure your well-intentioned words or actions hit the mark.

- Support her decisions. It's hard enough to understand all the nuances of mastectomy and reconstruction without having someone second-guess your decisions, especially after the fact. We all make decisions based on our individual priorities and fears. Respect your friend's decisions, even if you disagree with her.

- Don't avoid all contact because you feel awkward or you're nervous about saying the wrong thing. No matter what's going on in your life at the time, your absence or silence might make it seem as though you don't care or aren't interested, and that may strain your relationship. If you're tongue-tied around your friend and don't know what to say, tell her you're sorry she has to go through this experience and that you're there for her when she needs you. Or simply ask, "How are you doing today?" All conversation doesn't need to revolve around reconstruction and recovery. Talk about the weather, what the kids are up to, or what's going on in the neighborhood—the things you would discuss under other circumstances.

- Temper your contact, avoiding repeated phone calls or text messages throughout the day. Of course, never show up unannounced—your friend may love a visit, but on some days, she may not be up to it.

- Try not to be squeamish about surgical details your friend would like to share. Breast reconstruction isn't pretty at first. Try not to grimace or gasp as she explains her procedure in graphic detail, opens her shirt to show you her drains, or wants you to see her incisions. Inquire about her surgery, if you're curious, and then respect the extent to which she does or doesn't want to share.

- Make eye contact. Sometimes people feel so uncomfortable around recovering friends that they're embarrassed to look them in the eye. Even if you feel nervous, maintaining eye contact will show your friend that she has your undivided attention.

- Be sensitive to the situation. You probably know of others who have had cancer, and you may know of other women who have had reconstruction, but try to avoid comments such as:

"A co-worker had reconstruction a year ago and she's still in pain."
"Why on earth would you go through all that?"
"My aunt had breast cancer, too, and she died."
"I still don't understand why you just didn't have a lumpectomy."
"I can't imagine why you would choose to remove your breasts
    when you may never develop cancer."

Notes

CHAPTER 1. WHY MASTECTOMY?

1. Olson JS. *Bathsheba's Breast: Women, Cancer and History.* (Baltimore: Johns Hopkins University Press, 2005).

2. American Cancer Society. *Breast Cancer Facts & Figures 2015–2016.* www.cancer.org/acs/groups/content/@research/documents/document/acspc-046381.pdf.

3. Early Breast Cancer Trialists' Collaborative Group (EBCTCG). "Effect of radiotherapy after breast-conserving surgery on 10-year recurrence and 15-year breast cancer death: meta-analysis of individual patient data for 10,801 women in 17 randomised trials." *Lancet* 378, no. 9804 (2011): 1707–16.

4. Lyman GH, Temin S, Edge SB, et al. "Sentinel lymph node biopsy for patients with early-stage breast cancer: American Society of Clinical Oncology Clinical Practice Guideline Update." *Journal of Clinical Oncology* 32, no. 13 (2014): 1365–83.

5. American Cancer Society, "Surgery for breast cancer—axillary lymph node dissection." http://www.cancer.org/cancer/breastcancer/detailedguide/breast-cancer-treating-lymph-node-surgery.

6. Donker M, van Tienhoven G, Straver ME, et al. "Radiotherapy or surgery of the axilla after a positive sentinel node in breast cancer (EORTC 10981-22023 AMAROS): a randomized, multicentre, open-label, phase 3 non-inferiority trial." *Lancet Oncology* 15, no. 12 (2014): 1303–10.

7. Kummerow KL, Du L, Penson DF, et al. "Nationwide trends in mastectomy for early-stage breast cancer." *Journal of the American Medical Association Surgery* 150, no. 1 (2015): 9–16.

8. Smith GL, Ying X, Ya-Chen TS, et al. "Breast-conserving surgery in older patients with invasive breast cancer: current patterns of treatment across the United States." *Journal of the American College of Surgeons* 209, no. 4 (2009): 425–33.

9. Yi M, Meric-Bernstam F, Middleton LP, et al. "Predictors of contralateral breast cancer in patients with unilateral breast cancer undergoing contralateral prophylactic mastectomy." *Cancer* 115, no. 5 (2009): 962–71.

10. Wong SM, Freedman RA, Sagara Y, et al. "Growing use of contralateral prophylactic mastectomy despite no improvement in long-term survival for

invasive breast cancer." *Annals of Surgery,* March 2016. Epub prior to print; http://journals.lww.com/annalsofsurgery/Citation/publishahead/Growing_Use_of _Contralateral_Prophylactic.96963.aspx.

11. Sorbero ME, Dick AW, Beckjord EB, et al. "Diagnostic breast magnetic resonance imaging and contralateral prophylactic mastectomy." *Annals of Surgical Oncology* 16, no. 6 (2009):1597–605.

CHAPTER 3. BREAST RECONSTRUCTION BASICS

1. Santosa KB, Qi J, Kim HM, et al. "Effect of patient age on outcomes in breast reconstruction: results from a multicenter prospective study." *Journal of the American College of Surgeons.* Epub prior to print; http://dx.doi.org/10.1016/j .jamcollsurg.2016.09.003.

2. Song D, Slater K, Papsdorf M, et al. "Autologous breast reconstruction in women older than 65 years versus women younger than 65 years: a multi-center analysis." *Annals of Plastic Surgery* 76, no. 2 (2016): 155–63; Butz DR, Lapin B, Yao K, et al. "Advanced age is a predictor of 30-day complications after autologous but not implant-based postmastectomy breast reconstruction." *Plastic and Reconstructive Surgery* 135, no. 2 (2015): 253e–61e.

3. Qin C, Vaca E, Lovecchio F, et al. "Differential impact of non-insulin-dependent diabetes mellitus and insulin-dependent diabetes mellitus on breast reconstruction outcomes." *Breast Cancer Research and Treatment* 146, no. 2 (2014): 429–38.

4. Fischer JP, Nelson JA, Kovach SJ, et al. "Impact of obesity on outcomes in breast reconstruction: analysis of 15,937 patients from the ACS-NSQIP Datasets." *Journal of the American College of Surgeons* 217, no. 4 (2013): 656–64.

5. Alderman AK, Collins ED, Schott A, et al. "The impact of breast reconstruction on the delivery of chemotherapy." *Cancer* 116, no. 7 (2010): 1791–800; Harmeling JX, Kouwenberg CAE, Bijlard E, et al. "The effect of immediate breast reconstruction on the timing of adjuvant chemotherapy: a systematic review." *Breast Cancer Research and Treatment* 153, no. 2 (2015): 241–51.

6. Salgarello M, Visconti G, and Barone-Adesi L. "Fat grafting and breast reconstruction with implant: another option for irradiated breast cancer patients." *Plastic and Reconstructive Surgery* 129, no. 2 (2012): 317–29; Sarfati I, Ihrai T, Kaufman G, et al. "Adipose-tissue grafting to the post-mastectomy irradiated chest wall: preparing the ground for implant reconstruction." *Journal of Plastic, Reconstructive & Aesthetic Surgery* 64, no. 9 (2011): 1161–66.

7. Clemens MW and Kronowitz SJ. "Current perspectives on radiation therapy in autologous and prosthetic breast reconstruction." *Gland Surgery* 4, no. 3 (2015): 222–31; Baumann DP, Crosby MA, Selber JC, et al. "Optimal timing of delayed free lower abdominal flap breast reconstruction after postmastectomy radiation therapy." *Plastic and Reconstructive Surgery* 127, no. 3 (2011): 1100–1106.

CHAPTER 4. HOW MASTECTOMY AFFECTS RECONSTRUCTION

1. Reish RG, Lin A, Phillips NA, et al. "Breast reconstruction outcomes after nipple-sparing mastectomy and radiation therapy." *Plastic and Reconstructive Surgery* 135, no. 4 (2015): 959–66.

2. Stolier AJ and Wang J. "Terminal duct lobular units are scarce in the nipple: implications for prophylactic nipple-sparing mastectomy." *Annals of Surgical Oncology* 15, no. 2 (2008): 438–42; Jakub J, et al. "Multi-institutional study of the oncologic safety of prophylactic nipple-sparing mastectomy in a BRCA population." Presentation at the American Society of Breast Surgeons 17th Annual Meeting; April 13–18, 2016.

3. De La Cruz L, Moody AM, Tappy EE, et al. "Overall survival, disease-free survival, local recurrence, and nipple-areolar recurrence in the setting of nipple-sparing mastectomy: a meta-analysis and systematic review." *Annals of Surgical Oncology* 22, no. 10 (2015): 3241–49.

4. DellaCroce FJ, Blum CA, Sullivan SK, et al. "Nipple-sparing mastectomy and ptosis: perforator flap breast reconstruction allows full secondary mastopexy with complete nipple areolar repositioning." *Plastic and Reconstructive Surgery* 136, no. 1 (2015): 1e–9e.

CHAPTER 5. CONSIDERING PROPHYLACTIC MASTECTOMY

1. Antoniou A, Pharoah PD, Narod S, et al. "Average risks of breast and ovarian cancer associated with BRCA1 or BRCA2 mutations detected in case series unselected for family history: a combined analysis of 22 studies." *American Journal of Human Genetics* 72, no. 5 (2003): 1117–30; Chen S and Parmigiani G. "Meta-analysis of BRCA1 and BRCA2 penetrance." *Journal of Clinical Oncology* 25, no. 11 (2007): 1329–33.

2. Litton JK, Ready K, Chen H, et al. "Earlier age of onset of BRCA mutation-related cancers in subsequent generations." *Cancer* 118, no. 2 (2012): 321–25.

3. Rebbeck TR, Friebel T, Lynch HT, et al. "Bilateral prophylactic mastectomy reduces breast cancer risk in BRCA1 and BRCA2 mutation carriers: the PROSE Study Group." *Journal of Clinical Oncology* 22, no. 6 (2004): 1055–62.

4. Rebbeck TR, Kauff ND, and Domchek SM. "Meta-analysis of risk reduction estimates associated with risk-reducing salpingo-oophorectomy in BRCA1 or BRCA2 mutation carriers." *Journal of the National Cancer Institute* 101, no. 2 (2009): 80–87.

5. Rebbeck TR, Lynch HT, Neuhausen SL, et al. "Prophylactic oophorectomy in carriers of BRCA1 or BRCA2 mutations." *New England Journal of Medicine* 346, no. 21 (2002): 1616–22.

CHAPTER 6. BREAST IMPLANTS

1. American Society of Plastic Surgeons. "2015 reconstructive breast procedures." www.plasticsurgery.org/Documents/news-resources/statistics/2015 -statistics/reconstructive-breast-procedures-age.pdf.

2. Doren EL, Pierpont YN, Shivers SC, et al. "Comparison of Allergan, Mentor, and Sientra contoured cohesive gel breast implants: a single surgeon's 10-year experience." *Plastic and Reconstructive Surgery* 136, no. 5 (2015): 957–66; McCarthy CM, Klassen AF, Cano SJ, et al. "Patient satisfaction with postmastectomy breast reconstruction." *Cancer* 116, no. 24 (2010): 5584–91.

3. Institute of Medicine (US) Committee on the Safety of Silicone Breast Implants; Bondurant S, Ernster V, Herdman R, editors. *Safety of Silicone Breast Implants* (Washington, DC: National Academies Press, 1999).

4. U.S. Food and Drug Administration. "Anaplastic large cell lymphoma (ALCL)." www.fda.gov/medicaldevices/productsandmedicalprocedures/implantsandprosthe tics/breastimplants/ucm239995.htm.

5. American Society of Plastic Surgeons. "2015 reconstructive breast procedures." www.plasticsurgery.org.

6. Winocour S, Martinez-Jorge J, Habermann E, et al. "Early surgical site infection following tissue expander breast reconstruction with or without acellular dermal matrix: national benchmarking using National Surgical Quality Improvement Program." *Archives of Plastic Surgery* 42, no. 2 (2015): 194–200.

7. Salzberg CA, Ashikari AY, Berry C, et al. "Acellular matrix-assisted direct-to-implant breast reconstruction and capsular contracture: a 13-year experience." *Plastic and Reconstructive Surgery* 138, no. 2 (2016): 329–37; Namnoum JD and Moyer HR. "The role of acellular dermal matrix in the treatment of capsular contracture." *Clinics in Plastic Surgery* 39, no. 2 (2012): 127–36.

8. Moyer H, Ghazi B, and Losken A. "The effect of silicone gel bleed on capsular contracture: a generational study." *Plastic and Reconstructive Surgery* 130, no. 4 (2012): 793–800.

9. *FDA Update on the Safety of Silicone Gel-Filled Breast Implants*, June 2011. www.fda.gov/downloads/MedicalDevices/ProductsandMedicalProcedures /ImplantsandProsthetics/BreastImplants/UCM260090.pdf.

CHAPTER 7. THE EXPANDER EXPERIENCE

1. Ascherman JA, Jacoby A, Alizadeh K, et al. "Aeroform vs saline tissue expansion in breast reconstruction: a prospective multi-center randomized controlled clinical study." *Plastic and Reconstructive Surgery* 136, no. 4 (suppl., 2015): 84.

2. Gabriel A, Champaneria MC, and Maxwell GP. "The efficacy of botulinum toxin A in post-mastectomy breast reconstruction: a pilot study." *Aesthetic Surgery Journal* 35, no. 4 (2015): 402–9.

CHAPTER 8. TUMMY TUCK FLAPS

1. Chai SC, Umayaal S, and Saad AZ. "Successful pregnancy 'during' pedicled transverse rectus abdominis musculocutaneous flap for breast reconstruction with normal vaginal delivery." *Indian Journal of Plastic Surgery* 48, no. 1 (2015): 81–84.

2. Macadam S, Zhong T, Weichman K, et al. "Quality of life and patient-reported outcomes in breast cancer survivors: a multicenter comparison of four abdominally based autologous reconstruction methods." *Plastic and Reconstructive Surgery* 137, no. 3 (2016): 758–71.

3. Rao S, Stolle EC, Sher S, et al. "A multiple logistic regression analysis of complications following microsurgical breast reconstruction." *Gland Surgery* 3, no. 4 (2014): 226–31; Chang DW, Wang B, Robb GL, et al. "Effect of obesity on flap and donor-site complications in free transverse rectus abdominis myocutaneous flap breast reconstruction." *Plastic and Reconstructive Surgery* 105, no. 5 (2000): 1640–48.

CHAPTER 9. OTHER FLAP METHODS

1. Disa JJ, McCarthy CM, Mehrara BJ, et al. "Immediate latissimus dorsi/prosthetic breast reconstruction following salvage mastectomy after failed lumpectomy/irradiation." *Plastic and Reconstructive Surgery* 121, no. 4 (2008): 159e–64e.

2. Saint-Cyr M, Nagarkar P, Schaverien M, et al. "The pedicled descending branch muscle-sparing latissimus dorsi flap for breast reconstruction." *Plastic and Reconstructive Surgery* 123, no. 1 (2009): 13–24.

3. DellaCroce FJ and Sullivan SK. "Application and refinement of the superior gluteal artery perforator free flap for bilateral simultaneous breast reconstruction." *Plastic and Reconstructive Surgery* 116, no. 1 (2005): 97–103.

4. Saint-Cyr M, Shirvani A, and Wong C. "The transverse upper gracilis flap for breast reconstruction following liposuction of the thigh." *Microsurgery* 30, no. 8 (2010): 636–38.

CHAPTER 10. FIXES WITH FAT

1. American Society of Plastic Surgeons. *2012 Post-Mastectomy Fat Graft/Fat Transfer ASPS Guiding Principles.* www.plasticsurgery.org/Documents/Health-Policy/Principles/principle-2015-post-mastectomy-fat-grafting.pdf.

2. Panettiere P, Marchetti L, and Accorsi D. "The serial free fat transfer in irradiated prosthetic breast reconstructions." *Aesthetic Plastic Surgery* 33, no 5 (2009): 695–700.

3. Salgarello M, Visconti G, and Barone-Adesi, L. "Fat grafting and breast reconstruction with implant: another option for irradiated breast cancer Patients." *Plastic and Reconstructive Surgery* 129, no. 2 (2012): 317–29.

4. Charvet HJ, Orbay H, Wong MS, et al. "The oncologic safety of breast fat grafting and contradictions between basic science and clinical studies: a systematic review of the recent literature." *Annals of Plastic Surgery* 75, no. 4 (2015): 471–79.

5. Kronowitz SJ, Mandujano CC, Liu J, et al. "Lipofilling of the breast does not increase the risk of recurrence of breast cancer: a matched controlled study." *Plastic and Reconstructive Surgery* 137, no. 2 (2016): 385–93.

CHAPTER 11. ALTERING YOUR OPPOSITE BREAST

1. Charvet HJ, et al. "The oncologic safety of breast fat grafting and contradictions between basic science and clinical studies: a systematic review of the recent literature." *Annals of Plastic Surgery* 75, no. 4 (2015): 471–79.

CHAPTER 16. DEALING WITH PROBLEMS

1. Gdalevitch P, Van Laeken N, Bahng S, et al. "Effects of nitroglycerin ointment on mastectomy flap necrosis in immediate breast reconstruction: a randomized controlled trial." *Plastic and Reconstructive Surgery* 135, no. 6 (2015): 1530–39.

2. Matsen CB, Mehrara B, Eaton A, et al. "Skin flap necrosis after mastectomy with reconstruction: a prospective study." *Annals of Surgical Oncology* 23, no. 1 (2016): 257–64; Patel KM, Hill LM, Gatti ME, et al. "Management of massive mastectomy skin flap necrosis following autologous breast reconstruction." *Annals of Plastic Surgery* 69, no. 2 (2012): 139–44.

3. Loftus LS and Laronga C. "Evaluating patients with chronic pain after breast cancer surgery: the search for relief." *Journal of the American Medical Association* 302, no. 18 (2009): 2034–35.

4. Schmitz KH, Ahmed RL, Troxel A, et al. "Weight lifting in women with breast cancer–related lymphedema." *New England Journal of Medicine* 361 (2009): 664–73.

5. Gold MH, McGuire M, Mustoe TA, et al. "Updated international clinical recommendations on scar management: part 2—algorithms for scar prevention and treatment." *Dermatologic Surgery* 40, no. 8 (2014): 825–31.

Glossary

Acellular dermal matrix (ADM) Human donor or animal skin that has been stripped of its cellular material, sterilized, and used to replace missing tissue.

Adjuvant therapy Treatment given after surgery.

Anaplastic large cell lymphoma A rare type of non-Hodgkin lymphoma.

Anterolateral perforator Skin and fat taken from the front of the thigh to recreate a breast.

Areola The circle of darkened skin around the nipple.

Areola-sparing mastectomy A procedure that removes most of the breast tissue and nipple but preserves the breast skin and areola.

Asymmetry Uneven size, shape, or position of one breast relative to the other.

Attached flap Skin, fat, and muscle that remains connected to its original blood supply and is tunneled under the skin from the donor site to the chest to recreate a new breast; also called pedicled flap.

Attached TRAM flap Skin, fat, and muscle from the abdomen that remains connected to its original blood supply and is tunneled under the skin to the chest to recreate a new breast; also called pedicled TRAM.

Augmentation mammoplasty A cosmetic procedure to increase breast size.

Autologous reconstruction Reconstruction using a person's own tissue.

Axillary lymph node dissection Removal of underarm lymph nodes to determine whether cancer has spread beyond the breast.

Axillary reverse mapping A procedure that evaluates patterns of fluid drainage from the breast to the lymph node system.

Benign Non-cancerous.

Bilateral mastectomy Removal of both breasts.

Bilateral reconstruction Recreation of both breasts after mastectomy.

Bilateral salpingo-oophorectomy (BSO) Surgery to remove the ovaries.

Biopsy Removal and examination of sample cells, fluid, or tissue.

BRCA1 and BRCA2 (BReast CAncer genes 1 and 2) Genes that, when mutated, significantly increase the risk of developing breast and ovarian cancers.

Breast augmentation A cosmetic procedure to increase breast size.

Breast cancer Uncontrolled growth of abnormal breast cells.

Breast implant A device filled with saline or silicone gel that replaces missing breast tissue.

Breast lift (mastopexy) Surgery to reposition a breast higher on the chest.

Breast mound A reconstructed breast without a nipple or areola.

Breast reconstruction Surgery that uses an implant or a patient's own tissue to restore breast shape and volume after mastectomy.

Breast reduction (reduction mammoplasty) Surgery to reduce the size of the breast.

Capsular contracture Tightening of the scar capsule surrounding an implant.

Capsulectomy Surgery to remove hard scar tissue around an implant.

Capsulotomy A procedure that attempts to break the capsule of scar tissue surrounding an implant by compressing it.

Chemotherapy Drug treatment that destroys cancer cells.

Clinical trial A scientific study using human subjects, conducted to determine whether a drug or procedure is safe and effective.

Cohesive gel A viscous filling in silicone implants.

Collagen Connective tissue protein produced by the body.

Computed tomography (CT or CAT) scan An x-ray that produces sectional images of the body.

Contralateral prophylactic mastectomy Removal of the healthy breast that is opposite the treated breast.

Co-payment (co-pay) A fixed amount, predetermined by your health insurance policy, that you are required to pay for medical services or prescriptions.

CT angiogram Imaging technology that views blood vessels.

Debride Remove unhealthy tissue.

Deductible The amount you must pay out-of-pocket for medical expenses or prescriptions before your health insurance begins paying.

Deep inferior epigastric perforator (DIEP) flap Skin and fat taken from the abdomen to recreate a breast.

Delayed-immediate reconstruction Placement of a tissue expander to preserve breast shape and facilitate reconstruction when post-mastectomy radiation may be needed.

Delayed reconstruction Surgery to recreate a breast after recovery from mastectomy.

Delayed wound healing A wound that is slow to heal.

Delay procedure A minor surgical procedure performed before reconstruction to increase blood supply to the nipple or tissue flap.

Dermis The underlying tissue that supports the skin.

Direct-to-implant reconstruction Single-step reconstruction that places a full-sized implant immediately after nipple-sparing mastectomy; also called non-expansive, one-step, or single-stage implant reconstruction.

Dog ears Puckered ends of a scar.

Donor site A location on the body where tissue is borrowed to recreate a breast.

Doppler An instrument that evaluates blood flow.

Duct The part of the breast that delivers milk to the nipple.

Ductal carcinoma in situ (DCIS) Early-stage cancer that begins in the breast ducts.

Endoscopic latissimus dorsi reconstruction A reconstructive procedure that transfers the back muscle to the breast site entirely through the mastectomy incision or a small incision under the arm.

Epidermis The outer layer of skin.

Exchange surgery A secondary reconstructive operation to replace a tissue expander with an implant.

Extended DIEP flap Skin and fat from the abdomen and hip that is combined to recreate a breast.

Extended latissimus dorsi flap Skin, fat, and muscle taken from the back to create a new breast.

Extended transverse upper gracilis flap Skin, fat, and muscle taken from the inner thigh to recreate a breast.

Extrusion A condition in which an implant pokes through the skin.

Fascia The fibrous tissue covering the muscles.

Fat grafting Injecting liposuctioned body fat into the reconstructed breast (also called lipofilling).

Free flap Tissue that is transferred, along with its blood supply and a small portion of muscle, from one location on the body to another.

Free TRAM flap Skin, fat, and a small portion of muscle taken from the abdomen to recreate a breast.

Galactorrhea A spontaneous milky discharge from the breast that may occur after breast augmentation.

Gel bleed Droplets of oil that leach through the exterior of silicone breast implants.

Genetic Related to or influenced by genes.

Genetic counselor A health professional who is trained to interpret patterns in a family's medical history and estimate an individual's risk for disease.

Genetic mutation A change in a gene that may cause cancer.

Genetic testing Examination of a person's blood or saliva to determine whether she has a genetic mutation.

Gluteal artery perforator (GAP) flap Skin and fat taken from the buttocks to recreate a breast.

Granuloma A small area of inflamed tissue that sometimes develops around sutures.

Hematoma A collection of blood outside the blood vessels.

Hernia The protrusion of an organ through a weakened muscle.

Highly cohesive gel Semi-solid silicone used in some breast implants.

Hypertrophic scar A scar that rises above the level of the surrounding skin and may be painful or tender.

Immediate reconstruction Surgery to recreate a breast, directly following a mastectomy and while the patient is still sedated.

Inferior gluteal artery perforator (IGAP) flap Skin and fat taken from the lower buttock to recreate a breast.

Inframammary fold The crease under the breast.

In-network A group of doctors, hospitals, or other medical providers that are contracted with a particular health insurance company to accept predetermined fees for services.

Intercostal artery perforator (ICAP) flap Skin and fat taken from the underarm and used to fill out lumpectomy defects.

Invasive breast cancer Cancer that can spread beyond the breast.

Invasive ductal carcinoma (IDC) The most common form of breast cancer, which develops in the breast ducts and spreads to surrounding breast tissue; also called infiltrating ductal carcinoma.

Invasive lobular carcinoma Cancer that develops in the lobules of the breast and spreads to surrounding breast tissue; also called infiltrating lobular carcinoma.

Keloid A thick scar that spreads into the skin around an incision.

Lateral intercostal artery perforator (LICAP) flap Skin and fat from the side of the chest near the underarm used to fill out lumpectomy defects.

Lateral transverse thigh flap Skin and fat taken from the outer thigh to recreate a breast.

Latissimus dorsi myocutaneous (lat) flap Skin, fat, and muscle from the back that is tunneled under the skin to the chest to recreate a breast.

Lobule The part of the breast that produces milk.

Lumbar artery perforator (LAP) flap Skin and fat taken from the upper hip and waist to recreate a breast.

Lumpectomy Surgery to remove a breast tumor and a small amount of surrounding tissue.

Lymphedema Swelling in the arm or extremities caused by excess fluid after lymph node removal or radiation therapy.

Lymph nodes Small glands that filter impurities in the body.

Lymph system A network of small glands, connected by lymphatic vessels that filter impurities in the body.

Magnetic resonance imaging (MRI) A type of scan that uses magnets instead of radiation to produce images of the body's interior or detect ruptured breast implants.

Malignant Cancerous.

Malposition In the wrong position.

Mammogram An x-ray used to identify breast tissue abnormalities, including cancer.

Mastectomy Surgical removal of the breast.

Mastopexy (breast lift) Surgery to reposition a breast higher on the chest.

Metastasis The spread of cancer beyond its original location.

Microsurgeon A medical professional trained to perform intricate operations with special precision instruments.

Microsurgery Delicate surgery that requires special training and equipment to reconnect blood vessels.

Modified radical mastectomy Surgical removal of breast tissue, skin, some or all of the underarm lymph nodes, and the lining over the chest muscle.

Muscle-sparing latissimus dorsi flap Skin and fat taken from the back to recreate a breast.

Muscle-sparing TRAM flap Skin, fat, and a small portion of muscle taken from the abdomen to recreate a breast.

Necrosis Tissue or cell death.

Neoadjuvant therapy Treatment given before surgery.

Nipple banking A procedure performed during mastectomy that stores a woman's nipple in her groin until it can be later transferred to her reconstructed breast.

Nipple delay A surgical procedure to encourage new blood supply to the nipple.

Nipple reconstruction A surgical procedure that recreates new nipples after mastectomy.

Nipple sharing Using part of a healthy nipple to create a new nipple on the opposite breast.

Nipple-sparing mastectomy (NSM) Surgical removal of the breast tissue that preserves most breast skin, the nipple, and the areola.

Non-invasive breast cancer Cancer that doesn't spread beyond the breast.

Oncologist A physician who specializes in the treatment of cancer.

Out-of-network Doctors, hospitals, and other medical providers that aren't contracted with a particular health insurance company to accept predetermined fees for services.

Out-of-pocket cost The total amount you pay for medical services not covered by your health insurance.

Outpatient procedure A procedure that doesn't require an overnight hospital stay.

Pathologist A physician who determines whether cancerous cells are present in tissue samples.

Pectoralis muscles The pectoralis major and pectoralis minor muscles in the chest.

Pedicled flap Skin, fat, and muscle that remains connected to its original blood supply and is tunneled under the skin from the donor site to the chest to recreate a new breast; also called attached flap.

Perforating arteries Small arteries that run throughout muscle.

Perforator flap A muscle-sparing procedure that uses skin and fat to recreate a breast.

Periareolar Around the areola.

Periumbilical perforator (PUP) flap Skin and fat taken from the abdomen to recreate a breast.

Phantom sensation A perceived feeling from a missing body part.

Plastic surgeon A medical professional who specializes in cosmetic or reconstructive surgery.

Plastic surgery An operation performed to improve physical function or appearance.

Post-mastectomy pain syndrome (PMPS) Pain that persists after recovery from mastectomy.

Previvor Someone who has an inherited predisposition to cancer, but has not been diagnosed with cancer.

Profunda artery perforator (PAP) flap Skin and fat taken from the upper thigh below the buttock to recreate a breast.

Prophylactic bilateral mastectomy (PBM) Surgical removal of both breasts to reduce the risk of developing breast cancer.

Prosthesis A breast form worn in clothing to give the appearance of natural breasts.

Ptotic Excessively drooping tissue, as in a "ptotic breast."

Pulse oximeter A device that measures the level of oxygen in blood.

Quadrantectomy A type of lumpectomy that removes about one-fourth of a woman's breast tissue.

Radiation therapy Treatment with high-energy waves to destroy cancer cells and prevent recurrence.

Radical mastectomy Surgery that removes the breast tissue, nipple, areola, chest muscles, and underarm lymph nodes.

Re-excise Reopening a wound to remove cancerous, infected, or dead tissue.

Resorb To absorb again, as when the body reassimilates blood or fluid after surgery.

Revision surgery A surgical procedure to improve the results of an earlier operation.

Rippling Wavelike indentations in breast implants that show under the skin.

Rupture A breach in the shell of an implant.

Saline A sterile saltwater solution used to fill tissue expanders and some breast implants.

Scar A permanent change in the texture of the skin that grows over a wound.

Scar revision A procedure to improve the appearance of a scar.

Sentinel lymph node biopsy A minimally invasive method of sampling one to three lymph nodes to determine whether cancer has spread beyond the breast; also called sentinel node dissection or sentinel node mapping.

Seroma A collection of fluid under the skin.

Silent rupture An undetected leak in a silicone implant.

Silicone A synthetic gel that is used to fill some implants.

Skin graft Healthy skin that is transferred from one part of the body to another to replace damaged or missing skin.

Skin-sparing mastectomy Removal of the breast tissue, including the nipple and areola while preserving most of the breast skin to facilitate immediate reconstruction.

Spirometer A device that expands the lungs and strengthens breathing after surgery.

Stacked DIEP A combination of two abdominal flaps of fat and skin to recreate a single breast; also called double DIEP.

Subcutaneous mastectomy A procedure that deliberately leaves breast tissue behind during breast cancer surgery to preserve a patient's nipple and areola.

Superficial inferior epigastric artery (SIEA) flap Skin and fat taken from the abdomen used to recreate a breast.

Superior gluteal artery perforator (SGAP) flap Skin and fat taken from the upper buttock to recreate a breast.

Surgical drain A plastic bulb that collects fluids at the incision site after surgery.

Surgical oncologist A physician who specializes in cancer surgery.

Survivor Someone who has been successfully treated for cancer.

Symmastia Breasts that join together in the center of the chest.

Symmetry Breasts that appear to be of equal proportion, size, and shape.

Tattoo Pigment added beneath the skin.

Textured breast implant A breast implant that has a roughened exterior.

Thoracodorsal artery perforator (TAP or TDAP) flap A muscle-sparing flap of skin and fat taken from the back.

3-D nipple tattoo A tattoo that simulates the presence of a nipple on a reconstructed breast.

Tissue expander A temporary saline implant used to gradually stretch skin and muscle to make room for a full-sized implant.

Tissue flap An island of skin, fat, tissue, and sometimes muscle that is moved from one location on the body to another to replace missing tissue.

Total mastectomy Removal of the breast tissue, skin, and nipple to prevent or treat cancer; also called simple mastectomy.

Transumbilical breast augmentation (TUBA) Breast augmentation performed through an incision around the belly button.

Transverse rectus abdominis myocutaneous (TRAM) flap Skin, fat, and some or all of the abdominal muscle used to reconstruct a breast.

Transverse upper gracilis (TUG) flap Skin, fat, and muscle taken from the upper inner thigh to recreate a breast.

Transverse upper thigh (TUT) flap Skin and fat taken from the upper thigh to recreate a breast.

Unilateral mastectomy Removal of one breast.

Unilateral reconstruction Recreation of one breast after mastectomy.

Vascularized lymph node transfer A surgical procedure to replace previously removed lymph nodes with other healthy nodes.

Venous thromboembolism A blood clot that develops in a deep vein.

Vertical upper gracilis (VUG) flap Skin and fat taken from the upper thigh to recreate a breast.

Women's Health and Cancer Rights Act (WHCRA) Legislation requiring health insurance companies that pay for mastectomy to also pay for prostheses and reconstruction surgery.

Resources

BREAST CANCER

American Cancer Society (www.cancer.org)
BreastCancer.org (www.breastcancer.org)
National Cancer Institute (www.cancer.gov)
Susan G. Komen Breast Cancer Foundation (www.komen.org)
Young Survival Coalition (www.youngsurvival.org)

BREAST CANCER GENETICS AND RISK

Confronting Hereditary Breast and Ovarian Cancer by Sue Friedman, DVM,
    Rebecca Sutphen, MD, and Kathy Steligo
Facing Our Risk of Cancer Empowered (www.facingourrisk.org)
Informed Medical Decisions (www.informeddna.com)
In the Family (DVD), Kartemquin Films
My Destiny Foundation, Inc. (http://www.mydestiny-us.com)
National Society of Genetic Counselors (www.nsgc.org)

COPING

Breast Cancer Husband by Marc Silver
The Cancer Club (www.cancerclub.com)
Intimacy after Breast Cancer: Dealing with Your Body, Relationships, and Sex by
    Gina M. Maisano
Kids Konnected (www.kidskonnected.org)
Laughter Yoga (www.laughteryoga.org)
National Alliance of Caregiving (www.caregiving.org)
Prepare for Surgery, Heal Faster by Peggy Huddleston
Why I Wore Lipstick to My Mastectomy by Geralyn Lucas

INSURANCE AND PAYMENT ISSUES

Cancer Care (www.cancercare.org)

CareCredit (www.carecredit.com)

Insurance Information Institute (www.iii.org)

Medicare (www.medicare.gov)

Patient Advocate Foundation (www.patientadvocate.org)

The United Breast Cancer Foundation (www.ubcf.info)

The Women's Health and Cancer Rights Act (http://www.dol.gov/ebsa/publications
/whcra.html)

MASTECTOMY

Amoena (www.amoena.com)

BreastFree (www.breastfree.org)

BreastHealing.com (www.breasthealing.com)

The Breast Preservation Foundation (www.breastpreservationfoundation.org)

Flat & Fabulous (www.flatandfabulous.org)

Knitted Knockers (www.knittedknockers.org)

Nearly Me (www.nearlyme.org)

Reach to Recovery (www.cancer.org/treatment/supportprogramsservices
/reach-to-recovery)

Rub-on Nipples (www.breasthealing.com)

TLC (www.tlcdirect.org)

RECONSTRUCTION

American Society of Plastic Surgeons (www.plasticsurgery.org)

Breast Reconstruction: Your Choice (www.breastrecon.com)

Breast Reconstruction Awareness Day (www.breastreconusa.org)

The Cancer Survivors Network (http://csn.cancer.org/forum)

Facing Our Risk of Cancer Empowered (www.facingourrisk.org; search message
boards)

Food and Drug Administration (www.fda.gov; search for "breast implants")

Johns Hopkins Medicine (www.hopkinsbreastcenter.org/services/ask_expert)

Myself: Together Again (www.myselftogetheragain.org)

RECOVERY

American Cancer Society (www.cancer.org; search for "Exercises after Breast
Surgery")

Annie & Isabel hospital gowns (www.annieandisabel.com)

Marsupial (www.turnerhealth.com)

National Lymphedema Network (www.lymphnet.org)

Yoga and the Gentle Art of Healing: A Journey of Recovery after Breast Cancer (www
.amazon.com)

Index

Page numbers in italics signify figures.

ABOUT THE AUTHOR

Kathy Steligo is co-author of *Confronting Hereditary Breast and Ovarian Cancer* and *Confronting Chronic Pain*. A two-time breast cancer survivor, Kathy has twice had breast reconstruction.